WOMEN OF MAYO CLINIC

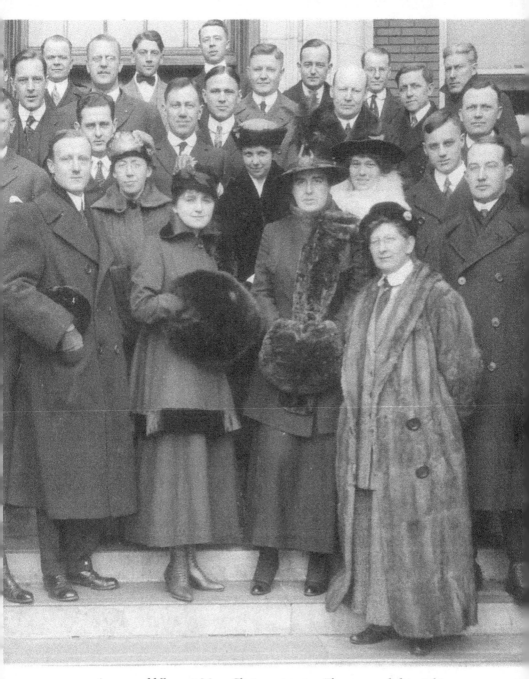

A group of fellows at Mayo Clinic, spring 1917. The women, left to right, Dr. Della Drips, Dr. Esther Owens (Ashton), Dr. Leda Stacy, Dr. Winifred Ashby, Dr. Dorothy Pettibone (Bruno), and Dr. Georgine Luden.

WOMEN OF MAYO CLINIC

THE FOUNDING GENERATION

VIRGINIA M. WRIGHT-PETERSON

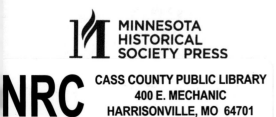

MINNESOTA
HISTORICAL
SOCIETY PRESS

The Eugenie M. Anderson Women in Public Affairs Fund

www.mnhspress.org
The Minnesota Historical Society Press is a member of the Association of American University Presses.

Manufactured in the United States of America

10 9 8 7 6 5 4 3 2

♾ The paper used in this publication meets the minimum requirements of the American National Standard for Information Sciences—Permanence for Printed Library Materials, ANSI Z39.48–1984.

International Standard Book Number
ISBN: 978-1-68134-000-5 (paper)
ISBN: 978-1-68134-001-2 (e-book)

Library of Congress Cataloging-in-Publication Data

Names: Wright-Peterson, Virginia M., author.
Title: Women of Mayo Clinic : the founding generation / Virginia M.
   Wright-Peterson.
Description: St. Paul, MN : Minnesota Historical Society Press, [2016] |
   Includes bibliographical references and index.
Identifiers: LCCN 2015037030 | ISBN 9781681340005 (pbk. : alk. paper) |
   ISBN 9781681340012 (ebook)
Subjects: LCSH: Women in medicine—History. | Mayo Clinic.
Classification: LCC R692 .W75 2016 | DDC 610.82—dc23
LC record available at http://lccn.loc.gov/2015037030

Front cover images, clockwise from top left: Maud Mellish Wilson, head of publications and library; Eleanora Fry (at left), illustrator; Dr. Georgine Luden, cancer researcher; Alice Magaw and Sister Joseph Dempsey in surgery with Dr. Will Mayo; Sister Joseph, hospital administrator—all used by permission of the W. Bruce Fye Center for the History of Medicine, Mayo Clinic, Rochester, Minnesota.

DEDICATED TO

Marlys, my mother,
who introduced me to the wonder of stories

AND

Kristina, Harper, and Heath,
who now share the joy of reading with us four generations deep

CONTENTS

INTRODUCTION

The idea for this book originated during Women's History Month in 2010, when a few colleagues and I working in the department of education at Mayo Clinic collaborated to create a Jeopardy game based on women from Mayo's past. When I visited the Mayo Clinic Historical Suite, I expected to find information on the few women I knew had been a part of the clinic's history. Instead, I was astounded to find name after name, folder after folder, and box after box of information on women involved in the very earliest days of the practice. I had never heard of most of these women, although I was born in Rochester and worked at Mayo Clinic for over seventeen years. I learned that several of the first physicians were women, and they started the laboratory, established radium therapy, opened a women's health section, and conducted cancer research. And there was a secretary, along with some Mayo nurses, who deployed with a medical unit to France during World War I. Other women played key roles in establishing the registration and medical records systems.

After the Jeopardy game, I looked at what had already been written about the history of women in southeastern Minnesota, thinking perhaps I had just missed learning about these women somehow. I checked one of the most comprehensive—or so it seemed—histories of the city of Rochester. I did not see much about women in the narrative, so I counted the photographs to estimate what proportion of the book focused on women. The book contains 270 photographs of people. Forty-nine of the images, only 18 percent, are of women. If that is not discouraging enough, I noticed that there are almost as many photographs of horses in the book as there are of women. And if the car had not replaced the horse midway through the narrative, there undoubtedly would have been many more pictures of horses.

At that point, I knew I had to write this book.

I have been on a fascinating four-year journey researching and writing. The stories continue to amaze me, but I encountered obstacles along the way. First, we do not collect women's stories, even unpublished, to the same extent that we retain men's stories. Men have historically been in the public sphere more through their vocations and military service. So they tend to write and be written about more, leaving more of a record. For every woman's story featured in this book, there are many, many more women who could have been included, but their names and narratives do not appear, or only minimal facts remain.

My intention is to provide a chronological narrative of Mayo Clinic focused on the most significant contributions of women without unnecessarily duplicating what has already been included in other histories, such as those on the Sisters of Saint Francis and Mayo Clinic nurses. In most cases, the stories and women included are representative of countless other women whose dedication and competence make Mayo Clinic the world-class organization it is. Once the nursing profession was fully integrated into the hospital and clinic practices, women began to account for 60 to 70 percent of the total staff and employees, a gender ratio that continues today.

In addition to a gender bias in recording histories, there is also racial and socioeconomic bias. Most of the characters in this narrative are white, middle-class women. I could find very little on women in lower economic circumstances. Sophia Tandberg Hogenson, the first "janitress" at Mayo Clinic, is an exception. Thanks to a remote mention in clinic records and information provided by her family, at least a portion of her story is here. But I know there are many, many more women who worked in entry-level jobs, making contributions deserving of recognition, whose stories we have lost. Also, there were very few women of color living and working in Rochester during these years, and I could find very little information about those who did. Again, I am grateful that we have some information on the first Spanish interpreter, Beatriz Montes, who came to Rochester from Havana, Cuba.

Depth, in addition to breadth, was also a challenge. I would have liked to include more of the personal, intimate side of all of these women. I have a sound foundation of dates, places, and actions, which is impressive, but I could not completely identify what motivated and sustained each of them. Relatively few letters and diaries written by these women survived them.

Nonetheless, these are powerful stories of strong, intelligent, and courageous women who persevered at a time when opportunities for women were limited. These women thought big and followed through with their plans despite barriers they encountered.

Quite possibly Mayo Clinic would have been very different if the men, especially Dr. William Worrall Mayo and his sons, had not been willing and wise enough to include capable women in their practice and in their personal lives. They were inclusive when it came to gender and religion. Perhaps these stories will help provide a more complete picture of the founding years.

I hope this book also inspires us to gather more women's stories, of the past and present. Although the extent to which the Mayos and their colleagues included women in the early years is unique, women have made significant contributions in other organizations and communities that are still untold. While current history books are more inclusive, many stories are still missing. Collecting the contributions of women today is important for having a comprehensive history in the future. We should expect the media, including local and national newspapers, to cover women equally. A quick count of photos in today's newspapers still shows a significant bias toward stories about men, although women are less likely to be outnumbered by accounts of horses and cars than they were forty years ago. More consciously collecting a comprehensive view of our own families and friends is important. Women and girls deserve an equal opportunity to be inspired by the stories of women.

Some of the stories in this book have been waiting a hundred years to be told; all of them reveal the strength, perseverance, intelligence, common sense, and talent of courageous women who were part of the establishment and early success of a world-renowned institution. I hope you enjoy reading them as much as I enjoyed the quest of finding and retelling them.

NOTE ON NAMES

MAYO PRACTICE AND CLINIC

The medical practice started by Dr. William Worrall Mayo and his sons Dr. William J. Mayo (Dr. Will) and Dr. Charles H. Mayo (Dr. Charlie) was referred to by various names in its early years. In this book, Mayo practice is consistently used until 1914, when the first building was built and Mayo Clinic was officially adopted as the name.

PHYSICIANS

The physicians in this book are referred to as Dr. and their last names in the context of their profession. When referring to them as husbands or wives or in personal matters, their first names are used. Dr. William J. Mayo and Dr. Charles H. Mayo were known as Dr. Will and Dr. Charlie, and this usage is applied in this book as well.

SISTERS OF SAINT FRANCIS

Many of the Sisters of Saint Francis were given the name Mary. To avoid confusion and for brevity, the name Mary has been omitted in this narrative. The sisters are referred to by their given names and their last names at birth the first time they are mentioned and then subsequently their given name only, omitting Mary. For example, Sister Mary Joseph Dempsey is referred to as Sister Joseph Dempsey initially and Sister Joseph subsequently.

SAINT MARYS HOSPITAL

The name of the hospital and its punctuation have changed over the years. For simplicity and to respect the last name given to it in 1968 by the Sisters of Saint Francis, the hospital is referred to as Saint Marys Hospital throughout this book.

ACADEMIC DEGREES AND PROFESSIONAL DESIGNATIONS

Because the names and related licenses of many allied health and nursing professions were emerging and changing over the decades covered by this book, and for brevity and clarity, none—such as RN—are used.

WOMEN OF MAYO CLINIC

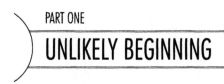

PART ONE

UNLIKELY BEGINNING

DISASTER STRIKES

AUGUST 21, 1883

More than a million patients from all fifty states and 143 countries arrive at the doors of Mayo Clinic every year seeking treatment for routine and life-threatening diseases. Facilities in six states with more than 4,000 physicians and scientists and 52,000 nurses and allied health staff collaborate to care for patients and assure that "the needs of the patient come first."[1]

The clinic began in Rochester, Minnesota, where the flagship medical center now includes two thousand hospital beds, twenty stories of diagnostic and research laboratories, and dozens of marble, granite, and glass buildings that appear like the city of Oz, rising out of the surrounding rural countryside. Shuttles move patients, specimens, supplies, and staff around a campus situated in the quiet city of 110,000 residents. The largest integrated private practice of medicine in the world, Mayo Clinic is among the top-ranking health care institutions. All of this began about a century and a half ago, inspired by a disaster and founded by relentless visionaries.

In 1883, Rochester was a twenty-eight-year-old rugged, aspiring prairie town nestled in southeastern Minnesota on land that had previously been a hunting ground for the Dakota. The Zumbro River, a tributary of the Mississippi, runs through it. The town began in 1855 as a stagecoach stop, when European homesteaders began flowing into the area. The settlers converted the oak savannas and prairies into fields of wheat, and agriculture quickly became the foundation of the economy. In 1864, the town's growth and prosperity was assured when the railroad came through, making it easier for farmers to get their crops to market. Churches, hotels, stores, and saloons sprang up along Broadway and the few cross streets.[2]

But on August 21, 1883, a sweltering summer day, while residents went about their daily business, a farmer paused from working in his fields just outside of town, a place that would eventually become the Rochester Country Club. He noticed the sky turning a strange coppery tone, and a ragged line of dark clouds began to shift in three different directions as gusts of wind picked up dust in the fields around him. Pelted by pebbles of dirt, he ran for cover as two dense funnels dropped from the sky and merged. With an ever-deepening roar, the massive cloud passed the farm and accelerated toward town, gyrating along the bed of Cascade Creek. The suction of the great cyclone pulled fish from the water and onto the banks while hailstones three inches in diameter and weighing a pound and a half hurled out of the sky.[3]

At the Franciscan convent on Center Street, a fourteen-year-old aspirant noticed the threatening weather approaching. When the girl's superior, Mother Alfred Moes, saw the greenish-bronze sky, she immediately called all of the sisters inside. They went directly to the basement and prayed hard, fearing the convent would topple over.[4]

As soon as the bank where he worked closed for the day, Mr. C. N. Ainslie, worried about the movement of the clouds and the changing colors in the sky, rode his high-wheel bike as fast as he could to the edge of town, where he knew the Congregational church was holding its annual Sunday school picnic, with more than a hundred children attending. Initially, the picnickers were reluctant to pack up, but Mr. Ainslie convinced them to leave just as the wind began to blow hard.

As Mr. Ainslie rode back into town, plate glass windows shattered and he overheard Mrs. Van Campen pleading with her husband to stay home rather than leave to check on the North Western Railroad depot. Within moments, the cyclone—a formidable force of destruction—descended on the little town. The Congregational church elders heard the rumble of the cyclone as they frantically shepherded the Sunday school children inside. They heard a thunderous crash as the church's steeple snapped off of the roof and fell to the ground, blocking the east entrance. The Methodist church's steeple fell too, crushing part of that building.[5]

Moments earlier Nina Cook, the youngest of nine girls, sat on the family's porch with some of her sisters and their grandmother. Her father, an architect, was out of town building grain elevators, and her mother and aunt were having tea at a neighbor's home. When the girls and their grandmother saw the sky turn a light green and then copper, Mamie, the oldest sister, urged them to get to the cellar quickly, which they all did, except for their grandfather, who was in the barn. The grandmother, a devout Methodist, prayed fervently for their safety while sand poured in around them and the storm raged above. Later, when they came out of the cellar, they saw that the second story of the house had blown off. They found their grandfather under a fallen barn door with his teeth knocked out, but otherwise unharmed.[6]

Their mother and aunt stumbled back home over the debris. The house where they had been having tea had been blown completely off its foundation. While the women had clung to each other in the cellar, an injured horse flew past, its entrails hanging out. When Mrs. Cook looked up, a piece of glass struck her, permanently blinding her in one eye.[7]

As the Cook girls' playmate next door ran toward a window in her house to look at the storm, a board crashed through the glass, impaling her and snuffing out her short life.[8]

As the tornado pressed through town, William (Will) and Charles (Charlie) Mayo were driving out to the slaughterhouse north of town in a horse-drawn buggy to pick up a sheep's head on which to practice eye operations. William had just returned to Rochester after graduating from medical school, and Charlie was home on break. Shortly after they arrived at the slaughterhouse, however, the skies grew dark and the butchers began closing up early to avoid being caught in the storm. The young Mayo brothers hurried back into town.

Just after Will and Charlie crossed the North Broadway Bridge, it fell into the river. The brothers watched as two grain elevators collapsed. When the cornice blew off of Cook's Hotel, part of it struck their buggy, freeing the horse. They managed to catch the frightened animal and take cover by a stone wall, next to the blacksmith's shop. While they huddled there, the wind peeled off the tin roof and crumpled it into a ball in front of them.[9]

The rain was heavy and the lightning constant as the storm took hold of the small town. Nearly twenty fatalities occurred instantly. The storm yanked an infant out of its mother's arms; it was lost forever. John M. Cole, a mill operator, was swept up by the wind and then thrown to the ground, widowing his invalid wife. The mangled corpse of a homeless man was found on the edge of town.[10]

After dark, when the wind and rain subsided, citizens lit kerosene lanterns and began searching the debris for survivors. The pinpoint lights of rescue parties bobbed through the wreckage. Fires broke out sporadically in the darkness, creating a dismal, apocalyptic scene. The injured were taken to the homes and hotels still standing and the German Library Association rooms. Forty patients were taken to the convent.[11]

Will and Charlie assisted their father, Dr. William Worrall Mayo, and other physicians in town as they tended to the injured throughout the night. They did the best they could with the few medical supplies they had. The deceased were taken to furniture stores until they could be transferred to the funeral homes.[12]

The next day the Rochester newspaper reported, "The work of the storm fiend is complete. . . . The death angel was enthroned about his dusky form, and together with a wild hideous roar, they swept down upon our beautiful city like a devouring demon. An hour later the pale moon beams fell upon a hundred ruined homes, a score of dead, upturned faces, and the night air was filled with the shrieks and groans of the wounded and dying."[13]

Long lines of relatives and friends filed through the undertakers' parlors looking for missing loved ones. Two sisters from the convent joined search parties. Rail cars were scattered about the tracks. An engineer who had jumped in an attempt to escape injury was found crushed under an engine. A twenty-year-old young man, possibly distraught by the storm, hanged himself in a barn. Crops had been scraped off the fields, barns were blown down, and scores of cattle, horses, hogs, and sheep were killed. Featherless chickens, otherwise unharmed, wandered along North Broadway. The worst of the damage was north of the railroad tracks in an area known as Lower Town, home to Rochester's working class.[14]

Oddities occurred during the storm as well. A heavy bed and dresser were blown across a floor and out the window while not a fork, dish, or napkin had been disturbed on the table set for dinner in the next room. Dresses were found hanging undamaged in tree branches forty feet above ground. Horace Leland's clock, found unbroken in the ruins of his house, had stopped running at 6:36, recording the exact time the storm hit.[15]

Mayor Samuel Whitten appointed a relief committee to begin assisting the citizens who were affected. People, bruised and cut, lined up for food, clothing, interim housing, and placement on a list for assistance in rebuilding their homes. Dr. William Worrall Mayo suggested bringing all of the patients from around town to Rommel Hall, a dance hall that could accommodate a large number and would allow the doctors to centralize their efforts. He

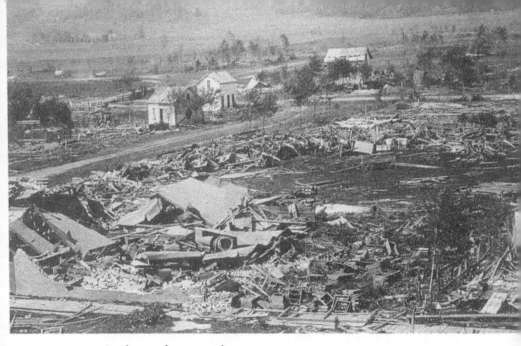

Rochester after 1883 cyclone

called upon Mother Alfred to ask the sisters to tend to the patients as well. Although the Franciscans were trained as teachers, not nurses, they learned quickly and provided around-the-clock care.[16]

Thursday morning, two days after the storm, was a pleasant summer day, but it was one of the saddest days in Rochester's history. Teams of horses pulling wagons gathered at Cook's Hotel to carry ten of the deceased to Oakwood Cemetery for burial, including an infant and five-year-old Nellie Irwin. The newspaper recorded the solemn occasion: "By noon the streets were crowded with a surging mass of humanity. The expression of sadness on every face, told more plainly than fluttering crepe or tolling bells the tale of mourning, desolation and death. . . . The ceremonies performed over the graves were very simple. No dirge was sung. No sound was heard but humble prayers and smothered moans of unutterable anguish. The only tributes left upon the close-clinging clay were silent, scalding tears."[17]

The storm left a path of destruction thirty-five miles long and up to a mile wide in places. Later categorized as an F5 tornado, the cyclone took more than forty lives. One hundred fifty families, more than five hundred people, were left destitute, homeless, with only the clothes they were wearing when the storm struck. Scores more endured injuries that would mark them for life. The flourishing pioneer town had been struck a brutal blow. Trees stripped of their bark and leaves stood bare with broken limbs, still reaching upward, signaling the city's great loss and deep despair.[18]

In the aftermath of the deadly cyclone, Mother Alfred quickly saw what was needed. Her vision of what *could be* expediently and formidably transcended the storm's devastation. She approached Dr. William Worrall Mayo about the possibility of building a hospital, which seemed ambitious given that the town had to rebuild one hundred fifty houses, as well as many farms, businesses, and schools. Dr. Mayo was reluctant. Such an undertaking would require a large financial investment, and even in prosperous times Rochester was much smaller than the cities that typically supported a hospital.

Dr. Mayo's reservations also stemmed from his nightmarish experiences in Bellevue Hospital in New York City in the 1840s, when he worked there as a pharmacist. Although somewhat improved, the conditions in that hospital were still deplorable when he returned in 1870 to obtain additional training after becoming a physician. Most people at that time believed hospitals were places to go to die, not places to be treated in hopes of recovery, and their concerns were well founded.[19]

The nationwide tension between Catholic and Protestant Christians posed another challenge. Although Mother Alfred and Dr. Mayo were not daunted by the differences in their religious beliefs, both knew it would require special effort to get Catholic and Protestant physicians to work side by side, and patients would not be accustomed to being treated by someone of another faith.[20]

And if these reasons were not enough, Dr. Mayo was already

sixty-four and Mother Alfred was fifty-four, ages when they might be expecting to wind down their careers rather than embarking on a bold, ambitious endeavor.

But none of these obstacles deterred Mother Alfred. She had thirty-two years of experience convincing men in authority, including a long list of friars and bishops. She promptly began raising the necessary funds. Dr. Mayo and his sons, knowing her capable and persistent nature, began visiting notable hospitals and drafting plans.

ARRIVING IN PIONEER ROCHESTER

1851–1883

Four women boldly found their way to Rochester in the mid- to late 1800s, when the town consisted of a few hotels, stores, churches, and saloons. Trains from the East Coast came only as far as Ohio, leaving prairie schooners, stagecoaches, and boats as the primary options of transportation into town. Jane Twentyman Graham, Louise Wright Mayo, Mother Alfred Moes, and Sister Barbara Moes followed different paths to Minnesota, arriving for different reasons, but their perseverance and contributions eventually served a common and extraordinary purpose. This is the story of Louise's journey.

———

"Good-bye, Louise. I am going to keep on driving until I get well or die."[1]

In the summer of 1854, Louise Wright Mayo stood at the door of her modest home in Lafayette, Indiana, watching her husband hitch his rig. After several summers of enduring headaches, chills, and fevers, William Worrall Mayo decided he'd had enough. Believing ague, also known as malaria, would be less intense in northern climates, he headed north, leaving Louise to fend for herself and their baby, as well as manage her millinery shop.

Malaria was prevalent throughout a wide swath of the Midwest, from the Canadian to the Mexican borders, and west to east from the Rocky to the Appalachian Mountains. Epidemics erupted among the first European colonists and spread across the continent for three hundred years until the illness was eradicated in the 1950s. Mosquitoes carrying the culprit parasite thrived in swampy, marshy areas and along the Mississippi waterways; Lafayette was directly in its path.[2]

Writers as well as physicians recorded malaria's presence and impact. Charles Dickens traveled along the Ohio and Mississippi Rivers in 1842 and described the town of Cairo, Illinois—about three hundred miles from Lafayette—as being "on ground so flat and low and marshy, that at certain seasons of the year, lies a breeding-place of fever, ague, and death . . . a dismal swamp . . . in whose baleful shade the wretched wanderers who are tempted hither, droop, and die, and lay their bones." In 1883, Mark Twain also described a favorite boyhood swimming hole along the Mississippi in Missouri, less than two hundred miles from Lafayette: "Bear Creek . . . was a famous breeder of chills and fever in its day. I remember one summer when everybody in town had this disease at once."[3]

A month after his departure, William had traveled nearly three hundred miles north to Galena, Illinois, where he recovered from his chills and fever. There he heard about the opening of Minnesota Territory. He bought a ticket on a steamboat headed to St. Paul to investigate the opportunities.

During this trip, William came in contact with a more deadly disease, cholera, an infection of the small intestine that can kill quickly by dehydration. It ravaged the United States intermittently from 1832 to 1873. In 1832, more than three thousand people died of cholera in New York City. Although lower economic classes were more susceptible to cholera due to crowded living conditions, the illness did not discriminate. Cholera claimed the lives of two U.S. presidents: James Polk in 1849 and, the following year, his successor, Zachary Taylor, who died of gastrointestinal infections likely to have included cholera.[4]

The Mississippi was especially contaminated, and William's journey upriver in 1853 was treacherous. He doctored victims on board the best he could, yet the vessel stopped periodically to dispatch the deceased.[5]

Despite his dangerous trip, once in St. Paul, William was impressed with the descriptions of the vast forests and mineral reserves that were said to be plentiful in the northern part of the territory. A few weeks later, he returned to Louise in Lafayette and suggested that they move to St. Paul because of the expanding opportunities there. Louise agreed, and in October 1853 they packed a covered wagon with their belongings and the remaining inventory from Louise's shop and headed five hundred miles north with Gertrude, their fifteen-month-old daughter.[6]

Louise and William originally met in La Porte, Indiana, in the fall of 1849, when William moved to town to attend medical school. Six years earlier, at age seventeen, Louise had traveled from her birthplace, Jordan, New York, to southeastern Michigan, where her aunt and two uncles lived. Her father died when she was very young, leaving her mother to raise three children. Louise made the trip alone, taking canal scows and prairie schooners. When her two uncles decided to move to La Porte, twenty miles away, she went with them.

Louise was smitten by William Worrall Mayo's English accent and by his strong presence—although he was only five foot four, a bit shorter than she was. She noted his quick, intentional way of walking. Direct and almost blunt when he spoke, William was driven by a desire to reduce human suffering, a drive which may have originated from his experiences growing up in Salford, England, outside of Manchester, where the scourge of industrialization of the sort described by Charles Dickens in *Oliver Twist* (1838) prevailed.

William had immigrated to the United States three years before he and Louise met. His father, a carpenter, died when William was seven years old. At fourteen, William apprenticed himself to a tailor, where he worked for seven years, attending evening classes taught by the Quaker tutor and famous scientist John Dalton. Dalton inspired William's love of the sciences. The Quakers educated women and men at a time when the Church of England only taught boys. Taking classes alongside female students may have contributed to William's appreciation for intelligent, capable women.

At twenty-one, William opened his own tailor shop, where he continued to work until July 19, 1846, the day he somewhat impulsively boarded a ship bound for the United States. He initially worked in the pharmacy at Bellevue Hospital in New York City. The conditions there were horrific; infectious diseases spread rampantly. Shortly after William arrived, ten of the thirteen physicians on staff died of typhus. William left and headed west, eventually making his way to Lafayette, Indiana, where he joined two tailors in business. In 1849, his fascination with science compelled him to begin medical school in La Porte.[7]

William graduated from medical school the following February and moved fifty miles south of La Porte to Lafayette, where he was employed at a pharmacy to advise patients. He and Louise courted long distance until they were married in the presence of family and a few friends on February 2, 1851, in Galien Woods, in southeastern Michigan, a forest so dense that it would be an important source of lumber for rebuilding Chicago after the fire of 1871.

Louise and William settled in Lafayette, where he continued to work for the pharmacy for a few months, until he went into partnership with another doctor in La Porte. Soon after their move, in November 1851, William assisted Louise in the birth of their first child, a son they named Horace, after Louise's father. Sadly, Horace lived only six weeks. The death of their child was the first of many adversities the Mayos would face throughout sixty years of marriage.

To help with the family finances and to fill the void left by the loss of their son, Louise opened the New York Millinery, on Illinois Street in Lafayette. She also took in boarders to supplement their income, supporting the family while William's medical practice grew. In addition to seeing patients, William and his partner began making and distributing medicines.

On July 18, 1853, Louise gave birth to Gertrude Emily; they called her Trude. The New York Millinery Shop was successful enough that Louise moved it to a larger location and brought in a business partner. A few months later, William's colleague was invited to teach at the University of Missouri Medical School in St. Louis. In November 1853, William decided to join him and acquire another medical degree, leaving Louise and their daughter in Lafayette.

By spring of 1854, William had completed his studies. He and his partner returned to their practice in Lafayette and collaborated on research on urinalysis, newly recognized as having diagnostic potential. They saw patients, although not everyone could pay them adequately. Louise's income continued to be an important source of financial support for the family during these years. All of this led to their move to Minnesota.

In St. Paul, Louise opened another shop, this one named the Fashionable Millinery, on Third Street, later called Kellogg Boulevard. For the northern climate, she added fur stoles, cuffs, and muffs to her inventory. However, William quickly determined that St. Paul had a surplus of doctors. Soon he was on the road again, leaving Louise to manage her store and care for Trude.

William spent the next year and a half exploring the woods and lakes of northern Minnesota. Traveling by foot and birch bark canoe, he made part of his living testing copper samples along Lake Superior. During these months, he spent time with the Ojibwe who lived in the region. Once he became lost in the wilderness, unable to find his way for days. Fortunately, some

Ojibwe men came across him and led him out of the woods. Yet another close call.

William's frequent and extended absences from home were not uncommon for men during the nineteenth century. A collection of letters written between women and their husbands in Little Falls, Minnesota, in the mid-1800s documents the challenges women encountered caring for a family, and sometimes running a business or farm, while their husbands went farther west in search of gold or a better place to live and make a living. Many men who moved west seemed restless and eager to avoid densely populated areas, like the father portrayed in Laura Ingalls Wilder's popular Little House series. Some men returned, collected their families, and took them to a new and presumably better place. Some men returned no wealthier, content to stay where they were. And some never returned.[8]

When William arrived back in St. Paul, he and Louise made a buying trip to New York for shop inventory. According to notes in Louise's account book, they bought more furs, including six "Victorines" opossum stoles. After the trip, her ad in the October 2, 1855, issue of a St. Paul paper read, "Mrs. L. W. Mayo is now prepared to supply all the ladies who may favor her with their patronage with the prevailing styles of the NEW YORK AND PARIS FASHIONS for Millinery and Dress Making. My Stock is replete with all the most exquisite can desire in a superior manner."[9]

Despite his wife's success with the store, William was frustrated with the politics of Minnesota's north woods and shore. He likely also missed practicing medicine. Louise and William visited friends they had known in Indiana who had moved to a place in Minnesota Territory known as the Big Woods, near the Minnesota River, a few miles from the growing town of Le Sueur. Coincidentally, Louise's uncle had some land in the area with a one-room log house he was not using. They decided to move there. William took their belongings upriver from St. Paul on a flatboat, while Louise stayed behind to reduce her inventory and find a buyer for her business.[10]

In May 1856, Louise, who was eight months pregnant, and Trude, now almost three years old, traveled seventy miles by stagecoach to their new rural home. Shortly after their arrival, on June 26, Louise gave birth to another daughter, Phoebe Louise. The move represented a significant turning point in Louise's life. For the first time, the family was living in a cabin located far from any city or village. Louise noted that their nearest "white" neighbor was fifteen miles away. Since she could not run her millinery business any longer, she turned her attention to homesteading.[11]

Pioneer women needed to make most everything by hand, including soap, candles, butter, and cheese. Often they raised nearly all of the family's food and would sell any excess vegetables or eggs for money toward the household budget. They milked cows, carded and spun wool from sheep they kept, and knitted and sewed clothes for the family. When the men were gone, they did heavier chores as well, including chopping wood, plowing, and slaughtering and dressing poultry.[12]

Soon after the family arrived in the Big Woods, Louise had an accident. Inexperienced at making lye soap, she was severely injured from inhaling the fumes when she tried to mix it in the cabin. This incident, plus the small size of their cabin, motivated Louise to begin spending as much time as possible outdoors, inspiring new interests and hobbies, including astronomy. "It was a rough, hard country," Louise recalled. "A few folk were comfortable, but most of us had to struggle to keep body and soul together."[13]

Meanwhile, William soon realized that there were not many patients in their area and most pioneers were accustomed to doing their own doctoring. He joined the local agricultural society in hopes of learning to farm. Ultimately, he operated a ferry along the Minnesota River to provide for the family.

While Louise and William were working hard to make a living, the world continued along its own course. A bank failure in 1857 caused a national economic recession, but Minnesota still became a state on May 11, 1858. The economic decline made land in town more affordable. Sensing that their rural location would not work for a doctor's office, Louise and William purchased two lots in Le Sueur in late 1858. On March 11, 1859, Louise gave birth to Sarah Frances in their crowded cabin. Weeks later, the Minnesota River flooded its banks, stranding the family because all surrounding trails were impassable and the river was too high and fast for William's ferry, further emphasizing the impracticality of their location for a medical practice.[14]

In 1859, William's brother, James, arrived in Le Sueur to help build a house. Despite the fact that their father had been a carpenter, the men did not have much construction experience. As a result, the house was built several inches off of square. Still, moving into town and into a larger home, even one not quite square, must have been a great relief to Louise. In November, shortly after they occupied the house, William's brother suddenly became ill and died.

Louise tended a garden, which helped supply William with herbal medicines as he turned his attention back to establishing a medical practice in town. She loved gardening and developed expertise in botany and the native plants typically used for healing: hyssop, tansy, yarrow, comfrey, and catnip.

Although William's medical practice was growing, he still needed another occupation to supplement his income, a reality common for physicians at this time. Building on his experience with the ferry, he became the captain of a small steamboat, transporting people and goods to and from St. Paul.

Trude, their oldest daughter, was school age, but the family endured another loss when her baby sister, Sarah Frances, died at eighteen months old. In eight years of marriage, Louise and William had lost two children and moved three times.

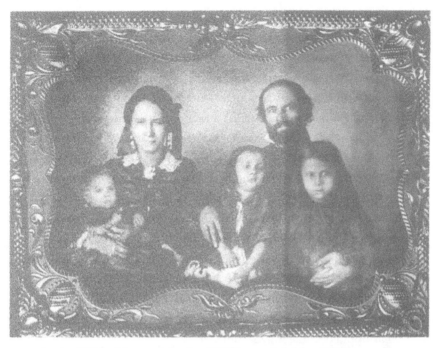

Louise Wright Mayo with husband William and children William, Phoebe, and Gertrude

to take his horse before the war broke out. Louise remembered him as one of "seven Indians who led the massacre, and who were hanged. . . . The Government gave his body to The Doctor, and it was from that bad old Indian's skeleton that my boys got their first instruction in anatomy. It hung in their father's office for thirty years. Before they could whistle they had learned the name of every bone in the human make-up from that skeleton."

It is not known whether William was given the body or he and other physicians took it and others after nightfall, as officials turned their backs, but the disposition of the bodies, the deaths at Fort Snelling, the relocation of many Dakota people from their homeland to other regions, and the bounty placed on any Indians who remained in Minnesota illustrate the violence of the conflict, which has not been adequately acknowledged and has thus evoked strong and conflicting emotions that have yet to fully heal.

As the violence in Minnesota waned, the Civil War gained momentum. The Union was recruiting soldiers. William was appointed as examining surgeon for the army on April 24, 1863, assigned to assess recruits in Rochester, one hundred miles away. He left Louise and his young growing family once more. Trude was nine, Phoebe was six, and Will was only two years old.

William was impressed with the booming town of Rochester, which had a population of 2,600 people when he arrived. A railroad would soon pass through the town, adding to its prosperity. William bought two lots on Franklin Street and hired people to build a log cabin for the family. His tenure with the army was short, and when Louise and the children arrived in Rochester in January 1864, William opened a private practice over Union Drug Store. After this, their fourth move, Louise proclaimed that Rochester would be the family's permanent home. They would not relocate again. Her firm stance set the eventual location of what would become Mayo Clinic.[17]

A year and a half later, on July 19, 1865, three months after Robert E. Lee surrendered to Ulysses S. Grant at Appomattox Court House in Virginia, Louise gave birth to Charles Horace in their modest cottage in the midst of the bustle of Rochester, on a spot where later the first Mayo Clinic would be built and subsequently a twelve-story Mayo Clinic building would stand.[18]

In addition to housework and childcare, Louise assisted William with his growing medical practice. In doing so, she contracted an eye infection, probably from one of his patients. Louise referred to it as "catching" sore eyes, most likely trachoma. She went "stone blind" for seven years, and yet continued to care for their home and children. No doubt Trude, the eldest, assumed considerable responsibility in the family during this time.[19]

In the fall of 1869, William announced to Louise—whose vision was still impaired—that he needed additional training in surgery and gynecology. He headed to Bellevue Hospital in New York. Although much improved from the time he spent there in the 1840s, it still had high infection and mortality rates. He left his account books with Louise so she could collect from patients who owed him, thereby supporting the family while he was away.[20]

When William returned from New York, the children met him at the train station. At home, while they enjoyed the special meal Louise had prepared, William mentioned the need for a six-hundred-dollar microscope. He had seen them in New York, and he knew how they could benefit his patients. The only way the family could afford the microscope was to mortgage the house. After asking for more details, Louise responded, "Well, William, if you could do better by the people with this new microscope, and you really think you need it, we will do it."[21]

In addition to this investment, Louise noted, "The Doctor had one weakness. It was for book agents. He knew and loved good books. Oh, many a time I planned to buy a dress for Trude or something for the boys or the house, only to have a book agent come to town, and kick over my bucket of milk."[22]

William was not the only one to benefit from the agents' wares, however. When her sight improved, Louise returned to reading books, including medical books. She frequently worked with William. He consulted with her on cases, and she assisted him with operations. Friends considered her knowledge of medicine nearly equal to his. When William was out of the office, patients would readily consult with Louise. Once, when she was walking downtown, she encountered a man in great pain due to a dislocated shoulder. She instructed him to lie down, placed her foot in his armpit, and gave his arm a pull, putting the man's shoulder back in place.[23]

During the first years that Louise and William were in Rochester, the city expanded. With growth came improvements, but also an increase in crime. Many immigrants to Minnesota were not prepared for the scandals and conditions they found. Wheat rings and railroad frauds cheated people out of their money. The Mayos not only supported their own family and community;

they also looked out for others, frequently taking in people who needed a place to stay until they got on their feet or returned to the East Coast or Europe.[24]

In the spring of 1873, doctors in St. Paul convinced William to relocate his practice there to be closer to more colleagues of his caliber as well as a medical school. Louise reaffirmed her commitment that the family would not move from Rochester, so William commuted while his family remained behind. The venture lasted barely a year. The practice did not prosper, and the commute was challenging and dangerous. William became stranded in Kasson on his way home during a snowstorm in the winter of 1874. Impatient when the trains stopped running, he decided to walk the eighteen miles back to Rochester, through snow drifting up to eight feet high along the railroad tracks. Soon after this incident, William returned his practice to Rochester, this time for good.[25]

In 1875, Louise and William purchased a thirty-five-acre farm just east of town. They built a large house, including a tower for Louise's four-foot telescope. She inspired her children with her love of the stars. Years later, her sons incorporated stargazing towers into their own homes, and seventy-five years later, the Homestead Memorial Church built on the Mayo farm site included a similar square tower on its steeple, illuminated in honor of Louise, the only memorial established for her in Rochester.[26]

Louise and William were committed to providing their children with the best educations possible. Louise said, "Only those who have good education can render the fullest service." She applied her practical experience in the garden to teach her children about botany, and when Will and Charlie attended private schools in Rochester, Louise took in boarders to pay for the tuition.[27]

Shortly after buying the farm, William left Louise and the family once more to spend three months in Europe to learn the latest medical techniques. By now, Louise was well accustomed to running the household in his absence, and the children were older and better able to help; Charlie, the youngest, was ten. And Louise, having a "strong sense of humor ... made thousands of friends in Rochester, many of them through her active participation in the doings of the Episcopal Church."[28]

At its Thanksgiving service in 1877, the Calvary Episcopal Church congregation devoted its plate collection to the "benefit of the sufferers by grasshoppers in the portion of the state most affected by them." Such generosity was sorely needed. Beginning in 1873, Rocky Mountain locusts had moved into Minnesota. Within hours of their arrival, fields of wheat were eaten clean. From 1873 to 1877, season after season, the grasshoppers repeatedly destroyed wheat, oat, corn, and barley crops. They laid their eggs deep in the soil, their offspring appearing the following spring. The grasshoppers came perilously close to Rochester, within a hundred miles, exemplifying the tenuous nature of farming communities at the time.[29]

On June 26, 1877, Louise and Will's eldest daughter, Trude, married Dr. David M. Berkman, a veterinary surgeon. The ceremony took place at the Mayo farm with the Episcopal priest officiating. Later that year, Mother Alfred and the Sisters of Saint Francis arrived in town at the invitation of Father Thomas O'Gorman. William had become friends and enjoyed conversations with Father O'Gorman because he was another learned man and because they often found themselves at the same bedsides of those who were ill or dying. Father O'Gorman wanted to have a Catholic school in Rochester. He initiated the fundraising, and by December, Mother Alfred and the sisters opened the Academy of Our Lady of Lourdes for students of all faiths. Initially a secondary boarding school for girls, later it also served as a day school for both girls and boys.[30]

The following year, Phoebe, the Mayos' second-oldest daughter, sustained severe injuries in an accident. She and Louise were coming home in a horse-drawn buggy when the horses began to turn into the driveway too sharply. Phoebe held tight to the reins and was thrown and then dragged to the house. She was badly injured and never completely recovered, remaining disabled for several years.

On April 7, 1878, Trude gave birth to Daisy Louise Berkman, the Mayos' first grandchild, who would later make her own mark on the Mayo medical practice. Two years later, on May 9, 1880, Martha May Berkman, the second grandchild, was born. That fall, Will left for medical school at the University of Michigan.

Louise remained busy. In December, she assisted Will, along with three other physicians, in one of the most difficult surgical cases he had ever performed, an ovariotomy resulting in the removal of a twenty-pound tumor. The success of this operation was reported in the newspaper, as was typical at the time: "Mrs. Waggoner . . . was doing well and out of danger. . . . The citizens of Rochester must feel equally glad that there is one amongst us who has the nerve and courage to undertake to relieve suffering humanity from this dangerous disease."

Although the Mayo children were growing up and leaving home, William brought home four more children after their mother, one of his patients, died. Members of the woman's family soon adopted the two younger children, but two girls remained with the Mayos until they married.

By 1881, Louise and William were living more comfortably than they ever had before. William's practice was successful and well established. Louise threw a big party for him on May 31, his sixty-second birthday, an event he described as the "greatest surprise of my life." More than two hundred fifty people attended, and the Rochester Cornet Band played. The community gave him the deluxe edition of Wilson and Bonaparte's five-volume *Natural History of the Birds of the United States.* William was quite touched by the community's expression of appreciation for his service.

After thirty-two years of marriage, enduring four moves and her husband's six extended absences, Louise was finally living a contented, stable life. All continued to go well for the Mayo family and the city of Rochester until August 21, 1883, when the community and many lives were changed forever.

PART TWO

WOMEN AND THE EARLY MEDICAL PRACTICE

OPENING SAINT MARYS HOSPITAL

1889–1897

After Louise Wright Mayo and her family arrived in Rochester and the cyclone devastated the town, Mother Alfred and the Sisters of Saint Francis worked long and hard to earn enough money to open a hospital. But Mother Alfred's story does not begin there. Her journey, and that of her blood sister, Sister Barbara, originated many years before, across the Atlantic Ocean in Luxembourg. They, along with Edith Graham, were instrumental in establishing the hospital, a critical resource for the development of the Mayo practice and which to this day sustains it.

———

The first patient was admitted to Saint Marys Hospital on September 30, 1889, six years after the disastrous cyclone hit. During those years, Mother Alfred and the Franciscan sisters worked relentlessly to raise the money necessary to build the hospital—giving music lessons and selling handicrafts they made in what little personal time they had after teaching and maintaining the academy and motherhouse, where thirty students boarded and twenty sisters and postulants resided. Their duties were manifold: they chopped their own wood, made their own soap, grew much of their own food, and spent as little as possible on clothes and linens, using flour sacks for pillowcases and buying two-dollar shoes. Each December, the sisters held a fair where they sold embroidery, needlework, paintings, wax flowers, and other crafts they had made during the year. The proceeds went into the hospital fund.[1]

After four years of extra work and saving, in July 1887 they were able to purchase nine acres of wooded land just west of Rochester. Dr. Mayo had chosen the location purposefully; he wanted the hospital away from the congestion, noise, and dust of the city, but still close enough to be convenient. When Mother Alfred brought the proposal to buy the land to the sisters, the decision was not unanimous; twenty-seven sisters approved of the plan and four voted against it. After ten years of working to establish a fine reputation in education, some of the sisters were concerned about diverting their energies and funds to health care. Some were worried that they were not prepared to be nurses; they had been educated as teachers.

Mother Alfred had a knack for convincing people. She went ahead and bought the land but made a much-needed three-story addition to the academy in Rochester before starting construction on the hospital, which pleased the sisters who wished to remain dedicated to their teaching mission. Still, many feared it would be impossible to raise the $40,000 necessary to build the hospital. But Mother Alfred persuaded the sisters at the congregation's twenty schools to save every possible cent. Ultimately, the hospital was funded from the schools' tuition, proceeds from the sale of some properties slated for schools, and money the sisters inherited, in addition to the funds they made from selling their crafts.[2]

While the sisters were busy raising funds, Dr. Mayo and his elder son, Dr. Will, traveled to hospitals in the East to explore optimal floor plans and lighting and heating systems. After several rounds of drawings, construction on the hospital began on August 1, 1888, and carried on through the winter.

The project faced challenges from the outset. Since there were few hospitals anywhere at the time, it was difficult to find an experienced builder. A few months into the construction, Mother Alfred heard a rumor that the contractor was behind schedule and might be planning to abandon the project. After some investigation, she discovered that almost all of the funds had been paid out to work-men and suppliers, but the building was only half done. Con-fronted with the prospect of having an unfinished building, just a stack of lumber and bricks, on her hands, Mother Alfred relied on her connections in the community. Indeed, the builder, whose most recent project had been a grain elevator, disappeared, appar-ently abandoning the job. A druggist and a banker in town were the project's bondsmen. Determined to assure that Mother Alfred's project would be completed, they forwarded the funds necessary to continue the construction while they tracked down the negli-gent contractor. They then helped Mother Alfred hire another builder to assume the job, and the project continued on schedule.[3]

Mother Alfred was actively involved in the construction. One day, Sister Cornelia Rappold, one of the aspirants, took mail out to the site, where she found Mother Alfred among piles of bricks, her skirt pinned up as she pored over the building plans. The sister noted not only Mother Alfred's intense engagement in the proj-ect, but that her petticoat was so completely patched as to appear more like a quilt than a petticoat, evidence of her frugal nature.

Finding Mother Alfred in the middle of a work site would not have come as a surprise to anyone who knew her. She was a tough-minded, immensely resourceful woman whose road to Rochester had been anything but easy. In fact, her life up to this point had been remarkable.

Before she was called Mother Alfred, Maria Catherine Moes was a new immigrant from Europe. When Maria and her sister Catherine stepped off a ship in New York City on November 8, 1851—the same year Louise Wright and William Worrell Mayo were married in Michigan—they joined twenty-three million European settlers and millions of Native Americans already in the United States. According to the ship's log, not all of the passen-gers survived the forty-two-day voyage from Havre, France; an infant and a twenty-four-year-old man died en route.[4]

Maria and Catherine's decision to immigrate to the New World when they were twenty-three and thirty years old, respectively, was probably influenced over time by personal, economic, and political considerations. Born on October 28, 1828, in Remich, Luxembourg, Maria was one of ten children raised by Peter-Gerard and Anna-Marie Botzem Moes. She and her older sister Catherine were confirmed on the same day in 1842 by a liberal-minded bishop, who overtly supported expanding the role of women in the church, which may have inspired the girls' choice of vocation.[5]

Although Peter-Gerard Moes was able to provide well for his family as an ironmonger, making metal fixtures, communion rails, and locks, the political and economic circumstances around them were crumbling. Nestled against the borders of France, Germany, and Belgium, the small country of Luxembourg had been under French rule until the fall of Napoleon in 1815, after which it became a pawn controlled by the Netherlands, Prussian forces, and Belgium at various times, creating uncertainty and a sense of instability.[6]

Luxembourg also experienced a significant decline in economic opportunity about the time the Moes sisters were born. In the mid-nineteenth century, improved hygiene and other health care advances caused a drastic reduction in infant mortality, and as a result, the population of Luxembourg grew by 42 percent. Although the enhanced health conditions improved longevity and the quality of life, the increasing population caused hardships in a land-based, agrarian economy. If a farming couple had eight surviving children, their farm was destined to be inherited by more people than it could support. In addition, Luxembourg experienced the same poor grain harvests and potato rot that much of Europe endured. By the mid-1840s, famine broke out. Almost everyone who set sail for the New World with Catherine and Maria listed farming as their occupation. Between 1840 and 1890, one in every six Luxembourgers immigrated to North

America. Products like cotton and tobacco were exported from the United States to various ports in Europe, where they were in high demand, and returning ships carried immigrants at reasonable fares to subsidize the costs of the return voyage.[7]

Before leaving their home country, Catherine and Maria received an education and learned skills that would serve them well in their varied roles in the New World. Initially educated at home, in 1842 Catherine and Maria began attending a convent boarding school in Metz, France, near the Luxembourg and German borders. They learned French, German, and a number of finishing school skills: needlework, painting, singing, and other arts. Maria was assertive, energetic, and confident, while older sister Catherine was more reserved, and perhaps not as healthy as Maria.[8]

In 1844, Bishop John Martin Henni, a Swiss priest recently appointed to the diocese of Milwaukee, traveled to Rome and throughout Europe to report on the church's progress and its needs, including a call for priests and others to join him in serving the church in the United States. Maria and Catherine likely heard him speak while they were in France, and his appeal may have contributed to their desire to immigrate. Catherine entered a convent in 1846; Maria was working as a domestic employee in Reisdorf, France, shortly before their departure.[9]

On September 27, 1851, passports in hand, Catherine and Maria boarded the *Caroline and Mary Clarke* in Havre, France, a popular port for immigrants heading to the United States. Before photographs were readily available, passports contained physical and character descriptions. The following narrative appeared in Maria's: "A meter and 650 millimeters in height (5 ft. 5 in.), auburn hair and eyebrows, high forehead, brown eyes, medium nose, ordinary mouth, and elongated face, healthy complexion, no disfigurements."

Catherine's passport included the following description: "A postulant in the convent of Peltre near Metz in France for the period of ten months . . . during her sojourn here has always been an observer of regular conduct, without the least complaint against her . . . a meter and 608 millimeters high (5 ft. 3 ¼ in.) black hair and eyebrows, low forehead, medium nose, medium mouth, rounded chin, brown eyes, oval face, healthy complexion, no disfigurements."[10]

The Moes sisters merged into American life at a time of unprecedented expansion, in stark contrast to the declining opportunities in Luxembourg. Millard Fillmore presided over a country with thirty-one states. Wisconsin, the sisters' destination, was the newest, its constitution having been ratified three years earlier. The national economy was growing, but tensions surrounding slavery were intensifying.

On November 8, 1851, the day of the Moes sisters' arrival, the New York Times, which had just begun publication a few months earlier, included articles on rising public concern about railroad accidents; a report of a patent dispute over the telegraph; and the announcement that a delegation of thirteen chiefs and two women from four midwestern tribes, including Dakota and Algonquin, were on their way to Washington, DC, for treaty discussions. The following week, Herman Melville's novel The Whale, later renamed Moby-Dick, was published—and promptly forgotten.[11]

A brutal winter was winding up when the Moes sisters arrived. In fact, in New York and across the young country, the winter of 1851–52 was promising to be one of the most severe of the nineteenth century, and must have been a startling contrast to the milder climate the sisters knew in Luxembourg. Despite the harsh weather, the sisters set off almost immediately for Bishop Henni's diocese in Wisconsin. Their exact route is not known. In 1851, trains stretched west continuously only as far as Ohio. Many immigrants took inland ships, but ice was a hazard in the winter months. Heavy snow frequently closed down the stagecoaches. Maps and guidebooks were not common at the time, and plenty of swindlers along the way took advantage of unwary travelers. Often, immigrants relied on letters from friends, neighbors, and family who had made the journey before them for descriptions of best routes and desirable towns.

Despite the potential for problems with ice, the Moes sisters most likely took a steamboat from New York to Albany, and then another to Buffalo before finally boarding a boat to Milwaukee, a journey that was probably not comfortable, given the weather and uncertainty along the way. In addition, Maria and Catherine must have faced a language barrier at times. They were fluent in their native language of Luxembourgish, as well as in German and French, but they did not speak English.[12]

In late November, Maria and Catherine arrived in Milwaukee, where they found a rich blend of immigrants from Germany, Ireland, and Poland. The city was also a destination for foreign-born Catholics, who represented more than half the population. Many of these newcomers were poor and had little formal education.

Almost immediately, Maria and Catherine encountered life-threatening health conditions. Animals roamed the streets of Milwaukee. Sewer and waste systems were rudimentary. Smallpox, diphtheria, and tuberculosis were rampant. A year before they arrived, a vessel known as the "plague ship" had docked in Milwaukee with three hundred passengers from Norway and Sweden, many of them infected with typhus.[13]

The sisters found Bishop Henni busy building parishes, schools, and St. John's Cathedral. He recommended the Moes sisters to the School of Sisters of Notre Dame, where they stayed until 1855. They did not take their vows there, however. The sisters had hoped to instruct children, especially Native American children, but because the new order was just being formed, it did not allow candidates to work outside the convent. Still, their time was not entirely wasted. Maria and Catherine learned English and refined their handiwork, embroidering church linens and making altar flowers, skills that were useful to them years later in raising the funds for Saint Marys.[14]

Determined to continue their lives of service, Maria and

Catherine asked to join the Marianites of Holy Cross in Notre Dame, Indiana. In 1856, they received the habit and were given the names Sister Alfred and Sister Barbara. At this point, the sisters were separated for the first time since immigrating. Sister Barbara was assigned to teach in Chicago while Sister Alfred was appointed to a school in La Porte, Indiana, seventy miles away. Sister Alfred was initially pleased to hear about her assignment. She assumed the state was named Indiana because it was the land of many tribes, and she hoped to be able to fulfill her dream of teaching Native Americans.[15]

During their time with the Sisters of the Holy Cross, Sisters Alfred and Barbara met a woman who became a powerful role model. Mother Angela, the mother superior of the congregation, responded to the dire need for nurses after the outbreak of the Civil War in April 1861. Sisters of the Holy Cross were among twelve orders, over six hundred sisters in total, that established and staffed eight hospitals and two hospital ships for the Union. To meet the need, Mother Angela retrained eighty teachers to be nurses, a practice Sister Alfred later replicated in Rochester.[16]

Sisters Alfred and Barbara were far from settled, however. Sister Alfred forged ahead on projects large and small. Occasionally her independent, unconventional style met resistance in parishes and communities. Sister Alfred was accused of favoring German students and charged with small infractions of conduct—doing what she thought best despite the rules. Subsequently, she and Sister Barbara were reassigned to a parish school in Lake County, Indiana.

Conflict within the Holy Cross congregations also emerged during these years. Some sisters desired to remain faithful to their French origins and traditions, while others preferred independence from French jurisdiction. As the divide widened, Sister Alfred took action. She sought and obtained approval to start a new Franciscan congregation. She, Sister Barbara, and two others from Holy Cross formed a community and were soon asked by a priest to establish a school in Joliet, Indiana. Sister Alfred, described as being "avaricious of time, with no personal experience of the meaning of the word idleness," was appointed the congregation's first mother superior.[17]

The sisters bought a small stone house in Joliet to use as their first convent. Due to the shortages of goods caused by the Civil War, they took in boarders and made crafts to supplement their income. People in town also supplied them with some necessities. They began a select school for girls, and between 1867 and 1872, more than seventy-nine women joined their ranks. The congregation grew quickly, opening six schools in Illinois, staffing a total of eleven schools, and expanding into Missouri, Ohio, Wisconsin, and Tennessee.[18]

In addition to the hardships brought on by the Civil War, challenges arose in unpredictable ways. The Great Chicago Fire of 1871 began within a few yards of St. Wenceslaus church and school, where some of the Joliet sisters taught. The parish buildings were not damaged, but Mother Alfred personally brought jugs of water and coffee by carriage forty-fives miles to the sisters living there. The congregation's archives recorded Mother Alfred's deed: "Unselfishness was one of her specific traits. She actually know not self, when there was a question of relieving those in need. The very best she was able to give, was not too good to be disposed of, to afford relief and comfort."[19]

Three years later, in 1874, when Mother Alfred and Sister Barbara's father died, each of them received a sizable inheritance. Mother Alfred made wise investments in properties, some of which generated rent income; others were sold at a profit. They also bought thirty-seven and a half acres in Joliet for a new academy and separate motherhouse, but the bishop stopped their plans for unknown reasons. Mother Alfred's independent spirit had not made her many friends among the bishops, who may have thought the sisters were becoming too autonomous and successful.[20]

The congregation had been asked to open schools in Waseca,

Minnesota, and Eau Claire, Wisconsin, and the sisters agreed that Mother Alfred should lead the projects. Although the bishop tried to stop her, Mother Alfred left Joliet by train and then took a stagecoach, beginning, at age forty-eight, a bold new chapter in her life.[21]

The challenges followed her. Mother Alfred and the pastor and parishioners in Waseca could not come to agreement about the location of the school. One possible source of the conflict might have been the Irish parishioners' discomfort with German-speaking sisters teaching their children. Undoubtedly Mother Alfred experienced a fair amount of discrimination in the United States due to her accent. Few people could discern between someone being of Luxembourgish or German descent, and discrimination against Germans started in the United States long before World War I. In the nineteenth century, nativist groups targeted rising immigrant populations, especially Irish, German, and Catholic newcomers to the country, believing they threatened American ideals.

In the midst of the controversy, a pastor in nearby Owatonna invited Mother Alfred to open an academy there. She accepted, and they opened a school in October 1877. During its construction, Father O'Gorman asked Mother Alfred to build yet another school in Rochester. She agreed, and only two months later, classes started at the Academy of Our Lady of Lourdes. Students of all faiths were welcome. Mother Alfred had an extraordinary talent for purchasing property and building and staffing schools in remarkably short time frames.[22]

The year the academy opened, Rochester—not even twenty-five years old—resembled a rough, unsophisticated hamlet with the challenges typical of a pioneer town. In addition to lawful, hardworking homesteaders, there were rogues and defrauders who took advantage of the lack of adequate law enforcement. Brawls on Broadway were not uncommon in the early years, and newspaper notices warned women not to walk in town unescorted.[23]

Despite the many challenges, some of Rochester's early citizens promoted educated dialogue. Two library associations and several civic groups brought speakers to town. On December 25, 1877, although "the weather was lowery and threatening and the condition of the streets and highways simply horrible," the nationally known woman's suffragist Susan B. Anthony spoke at Heaney's Hall to a "good and highly appreciative audience." She suggested that since emancipated slaves and Mexican immigrants had been given the right to vote, it was time to give the same right to the "intelligent mothers and wives of the country." With the thousands of petitions that were flowing into Washington, DC, she expected that the Sixteenth Amendment, conferring the right to vote on women, would pass soon. Unfortunately, women had to wait forty-three years from the evening of Anthony's talk in Rochester, until 1920, for the Nineteenth Amendment to be ratified.[24]

Along with the citizens who brought Susan B. Anthony to speak, the Rochester newspaper supported the woman suffrage movement in 1877: "There is no reason why women should not vote ... on all questions. Women have the same interest in government as men, and should have the same facilities for voting on all questions that men have. [The constitution] ought to be so amended as to allow them to vote whenever and wherever men do."[25]

Clearly, Mother Alfred was in a town of citizens who fostered progressive attitudes, fertile ground for the sisters and other women to make significant contributions to the establishment of an internationally renowned medical center.

Despite the auspicious start in Rochester, Mother Alfred's difficulties were not at an end. That same month, December 1877, the bishop in Illinois discovered that funds from his diocese had been used for schools in Minnesota, and he was not pleased. It is quite possible that much of the money originated from the sisters' inheritances and what they raised from school tuitions. Within weeks of the academy opening in Rochester, he terminated Mother Alfred's relationship with her congregation in Joliet and summoned any sisters who wished to remain affiliated with it to return to Indiana at once. Twenty-five sisters chose to remain under Mother Alfred's leadership, including her blood sister, Sister Barbara, who had been teaching in Joliet. Undaunted, Mother Alfred appealed to Bishop Thomas Grace in St. Paul, Minnesota, who authorized her to form a new congregation of Franciscan sisters in Rochester, allowing them to continue their mission.[26]

Over the next five years, from 1878 to 1883, the sisters doubled their numbers and opened schools in Minnesota, Ohio, and Kentucky, a testament to the perseverance and hard work of the entire congregation. Mother Alfred and Sister Barbara repeatedly demonstrated their courage and resilience from the time they left their home and family in Luxembourg, traveling from state to state, parish to parish. Yet perhaps the greatest challenges and opportunities were still ahead of them. They were prospering, until that hot summer day, August 21, 1883, when the cyclone changed everything in Rochester.[27]

The *Rochester Post* reported the opening of Saint Marys Hospital in its October 4, 1889, issue. Five patients were already being cared for in the three-story, four-thousand-square-foot, red brick building. The floors were maple with two thicknesses of felt between the wood and the lining to make them as quiet as possible. Wards sufficient to hold a total of twenty-seven patients were placed on the first, second, and third floors. The first floor also held the reception parlor, offices, pantry, and kitchen. The range in the kitchen had an eighty-gallon boiler that was the source for piped hot water throughout the building. A bay window and skylight were built into the twelve-foot-square surgical suite on the second floor to assure optimal light for operations. The chapel and sacristy were on the third floor, along with dormitory rooms for the sisters working there. The third floor was also home to a large recreation hall, where patients could exercise and access reading material during their stay.[28]

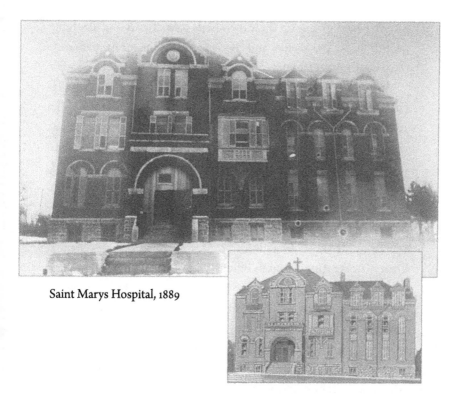

Saint Marys Hospital, 1889

The hospital was complete with modern conveniences. Running hot and cold water was available when it opened, and gas lighting would be added soon. According to the newspaper, the rooms throughout were large and well lighted and ventilated. Further, the article noted that "everything about the building is clean and new and every convenience has been provided to make the place pleasant and homelike for the sick."

Although the building was complete, initially it was sparsely furnished. The sisters made an appeal to the citizens of Rochester to help with furniture and linens. Sadly, few responded to their requests, possibly a sign of tempered enthusiasm for the hospital. They began with only a dozen iron cots, unbleached muslin linens, and rough gowns. They were given some "garish" quilts and some mattresses that did not fit the bed frames, requiring the nurses to be ever alert that a patient did not slide off the bed.

Sisters began giving up their own beds for patients and sleeping on the floor. The dishes and utensils that went up on patients' trays were mismatched.

While the fixtures were in place, the building did not initially have gas service, so the sisters carried lanterns through the halls after dark to find their way and left a lantern lit outside the front entrance for anyone arriving overnight. Anticipating the installation of an elevator, a shaft had been built, but it created a hazard until a safety rail could be added; one of the sisters sat guard in the evenings to prevent anyone from falling into it.[29]

At the time of the opening, the twenty-seven-bed hospital was staffed by six sisters in addition to Mother Alfred: Sisters Sienna Otto, Constantine Koupal, Fidelis Cashion, Hyacinth Quinlan, Fabian Halloran, and Sylvester Burke. A few weeks later, Sister Joseph Dempsey joined them after being reassigned from her position as director of a school in Ashland, Kentucky. These sisters provided around-the-clock care for the patients and were soon assisting in surgery. They came from farms and small towns across the Midwest, and although they were not trained in nursing specifically, Mother Alfred chose them because she knew them to be hardworking and resourceful. They covered all of the nursing duties, which at the time included cooking and serving meals, housekeeping, dressing wounds, giving medications, and keeping patients comfortable.

Their workday began at 3:00 or 4:00 AM and ended near midnight. They started with the operating room linen and made their way through the day's duties, ending with bedside care of patients. When patients required around-the-clock nursing, a shift of two days with an intervening night was not unusual.[30]

Mother Alfred was known for nurturing the spirituality of the sisters in her congregation in light of their long hours and hard work. She ensured that priests came in to provide spiritual conferences for all of the sisters, and she provided the latest ascetical books. They would read during meals and for half an hour in the evening, the sisters sewing, mending, and doing other handwork while listening to one of their members read. Beyond these daily rituals, they devoted one day a month to a retreat, spending most of it in silence and prayer.

Mother Alfred's favorite prayer was Psalm 37, which includes the phrase "Commit your way to the Lord, trust in Him and He will act." This verse must have been of great support and solace to her and the other sisters as they embarked on so many new ventures, often without any earthly assurance that their plans would work out. The verse may have been important in fueling Mother Alfred's persistence in the face of the obstacles and barriers she so often encountered. Mother Alfred also took time for reflection. She found happiness working in the garden the sisters relied on for food and flowers.[31]

Another characteristic of Mother Alfred's leadership was that she never thought of any task as too menial for her to do herself. She carried wood and helped with canning the garden's harvest, both tasks that some might consider beneath her position. She was recognized by many to be multi-talented: a competent teacher, musician, businesswoman, gardener, embroidery and needlepoint artist, organizer, leader, community contact, and visionary.[32]

Saint Marys was not the first hospital in Rochester. The Second State Hospital for the Insane had opened ten years earlier, able to serve seventy to eighty patients. The first hospital built for the mentally ill, in St. Peter, Minnesota, had reached its capacity of seven hundred patients. Rather than expand, the decision was made to start another hospital in Rochester. Coincidentally, the same day that the *Rochester Post* reported the opening of Saint Marys, it also reported the results of an investigation of maltreatment and abuse of patients at Rochester's Hospital for the Insane. Although superintendent Dr. J. E. Bowers was absolved of wrongdoing, he chose to resign. He claimed that of the two thousand patients treated during his tenure only ninety-six cases of concern were raised, and many of those were never brought to

Mother Alfred Moes

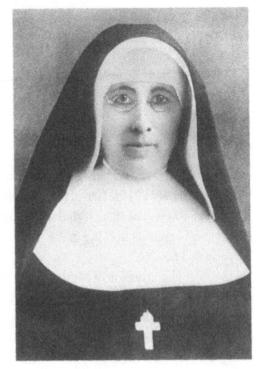

his attention because the attendants had a pact among themselves not to report wrongful acts. The governor's review committee made various recommendations about the hiring and supervision of attendants in the future. The publicity detailing poor treatment at a local hospital affirmed the relatively negative attitudes the general public held toward hospital care.[33]

In addition to public wariness about hospitals, the sisters encountered religious discrimination. When Saint Marys opened, it accepted patients regardless of color, sex, financial status, or religion. Mother Alfred stated clearly, "The cause of suffering humanity knows no religion and no sex; the charity of the Sisters of St. Francis is as broad as their religion." Mother Alfred chose to affiliate with Dr. Mayo because in her opinion he was the most competent physician in town. The fact he was an Episcopalian did not deter her, nor did it prevent him from committing to work with her.[34]

Although Mother Alfred and Dr. Mayo could see beyond the borders of their faiths, many people and physicians in town could not. Anti-Catholicism had increased between 1860 and 1890 as the Catholic population in the United States tripled. The American Protective Association, a predecessor to the Ku Klux Klan and the most vehement anti-Catholic movement in the nation, had organized 250 miles away in Clinton, Iowa, in 1887. According to one description of resistance to Saint Marys, "Ardent Protestants would have none of an institution that was managed by black-robed nuns and in which there was a chapel set aside for the exercises of popery."[35]

Appointment of a prominent local Presbyterian to collaborate in the superintendence of the hospital—an attempt to reach out to Protestants—actually made matters worse. Catholics who were supportive of the hospital resisted the involvement of another denomination in the hospital leadership. This concern was eventually alleviated when Joseph B. Cotter was appointed bishop of the Catholic diocese and expressed his support for Saint Marys Hospital.

Despite the discrimination, acceptance of the Catholic hospital eventually grew. Olmsted County began providing financial support for the care of its wards; the three Masonic lodges in town supported a bed for their members; and friends of the hospital held a charity ball. Protestant physicians began to use the hospital, some sincerely, while others began to dump only their most highly contagious and terminally ill patients there. This practice threatened the health of the patients and the sisters and drove up the hospital mortality rate. As a protective measure, the sisters insisted that all patients be examined by one of the Mayos before being admitted.[36]

If the financial and religious challenges were not enough, Mother Alfred encountered yet more difficulties with a bishop just before the hospital opened. In late summer of 1889, Archbishop John Ireland called for an election of a new mother superior for the congregation. Possibly some of the sisters had complained that they were being worked too hard. Some still might have been resentful about opening and operating a hospital in addition to their teaching mission.

Despite Archbishop Ireland's instruction that Mother Alfred's name was not permitted on the ballot, every vote was cast for her. He ignored the votes and appointed a reluctant Sister Matilda to be the mother superior. As the thirty-eight-year-old worked with her mentor, she appointed Mother Alfred superintendent of Saint Marys Hospital.

Mother Alfred recruited the sisters who would join her on opening day, September 29, 1889. She also had a sense of which sister would make an excellent leader for the hospital in the future. She began plans to have Sister Joseph Dempsey reassigned from her position as director of Holy Family School in Ashland, Kentucky. Mother Alfred had to make the assignment without upsetting the area's pastor or bishop. She cleverly asked her blood sister, Sister Barbara, superior of a school in nearby Ironton, Ohio, to be present at the annual confirmation at Holy Family on November 5, 1889. Sister Barbara verified that the bishop and pastor were pleased with the sisters assigned there, including Sister Joseph. Since the bishop would likely not make another visit for a year, it would be relatively safe to reassign Sister Joseph after that visit.

On November 5, Sister Hyacinth Quinlan, Mother Alfred's "trouble-shooter" and "reliable filler-in," left for Kentucky to replace Sister Joseph so she could return to Rochester for assignment at Saint Marys. Sister Joseph arrived November 19 and commenced her duties as a nurse that same day, the beginning of a forty-seven-year career, most of which would be spent at the hospital's helm.[37]

But Sister Joseph had no experience as a nurse. In fact, none of the sisters did. Fortunately, Dr. Mayo had hired Edith Graham, a nurse who had graduated from Chicago Women's Hospital in the spring of 1889. A local woman, Edith benefited from both her mother's extensive experience as a well-respected midwife and her formal education in Chicago.

Having completed her nurse's training, Edith returned to Rochester looking for work after her first employer, a doctor in Chicago, fired her on the spot when she reported for duty after being assigned to him by the school. He claimed she was "too young and too beautiful." Edith was twenty-two years old and five feet two and one-half inches, with brown eyes and hair. Dr. Charlie Mayo described her as "a radiant and truly beautiful woman." Luckily for Edith, the elder Dr. Mayo "was not a man to allow a woman's beauty to obscure her professional qualifications."[38]

Like so many of the women who contributed to the establishment of the Mayo Clinic, Edith's road to Rochester was a pioneer's trail. She had yet to be born in May 1856 when her parents, Joseph and Jane Twentyman Graham, loaded up a wagon in Cortland, New York, with their belongings and their six children, ages three months to eight years, and headed for Minnesota Territory. The farm they bought had a shanty house on it from the previous owner. It consisted of one room, long and narrow like a shoebox. A long drum stove stood in the middle. They hung their clothes on pegs along the wall and slept on cornhusk and straw mattresses on the floor. Soon, Joseph and the boys built a bedroom for Jane in a log addition at one end, complete with a wood bedstead. The little children slept on the floor in her room. The older girls slept in a loft overhead in the main part of the house, while the boys slept below. They also added a kitchen with a cookstove.

The Grahams had seven more children after arriving in Minnesota, bringing the total to thirteen. Edith was one of these children. On the morning of February 12, 1867, Edith's older brother Christopher "Kit" recalled being asked by his mother to go outside and cut large chunks of snow. She said she needed a lot of hot water to do laundry that day. After he had made four or five trips, filling a large pan on the stove, she sent him outside for more wood and then told him to go on another errand for her.

In his absence, Edith Maria, the eleventh of the thirteen Graham children, was born. Edith and Kit became close friends. In a letter to her on her sixtieth birthday, Kit wrote, "Nothing so important has ever made me so delighted in living. You surrounded my heart and have kept me thinking, challenged and solid all my life. You were the greatest gift, and what outshines even that—you have constantly and softly touched everyone I know."[39]

In 1869, the Grahams built a new house with a porch on the front. Life became more comfortable, but there were still challenges. One day while in the field helping Joseph bind grain, Jane was bitten on the leg by a snake, possibly a venomous rattlesnake. Joseph sent one of the older boys running to the tavern to get some whiskey. He poured some of the whiskey on the bite and gave her some to drink. Fortunately, she survived.[40]

Edith's parents emphasized the importance of education. The Graham children walked a mile and three-quarters to Kalmer Township District School Number 24, part of the Olmsted County school system. Two years before Edith was born, a new superintendent developed an innovative curriculum and several textbooks, which were used locally and sold throughout the United States. He implemented advanced teaching techniques in the very rural area.[41]

In 1880, when she was thirteen, Edith wrote an essay entitled "Women's Rights."

> Now, first of all women have as good a right to vote as men. And if every thing was as it should be they would vote. . . . The idea of women not knowing enough to hold office, where you see one smart man you see a dozen smart women. And to hear a man say a woman don't know enough to hold office, when he is scarcely more than a fool himself is ridiculous. And I say that woman who will listen to it don't know her own mind but ought to learn it.

I think a woman has as good right to be President as a man and would raise Congress right along if she could be Secretary of State or something of this kind. And I think it is just awful the way they have to make [women] scrub, milk, dig holes, etc. when they were born to something higher. But No, their brothers must have the education, he must work, he must be king if possible. He is a boy.

Yes, that is the way, but it won't be long if I can help it. Follow my example, girls, and we will soon vote, and hold office, be President, and serve in Congress."

E.M.G., Esquire

Despite her ardent argument and optimism, Edith had to wait another forty years, until she was fifty-two, to vote in a national election.[42]

After completing her education in the Olmsted County school system, Edith taught in the area until she was twenty years old. In 1887, she and her sister Dinah and two friends decided to go to nursing school at the Chicago Hospital for Women and Children, three hundred miles away. Undoubtedly, Edith's mother, Jane Twentyman Graham, had influenced them. Jane was a "woman of rare courage, deep religious faith, warm sympathy and a natural talent for soothing the sick and making them comfortable." She was an accomplished midwife, and her abilities to provide obstetrical assistance were considered equivalent to, if not better than, those of most physicians. Her children estimated that throughout her career she had aided in the births of 243 babies without losing a mother or an infant, a remarkable record.[43]

Going away to nursing school must have taken courage. Not only were the young women far from home; they were in the midst of a bustling metropolis. In contrast to a prairie town of four thousand people, Chicago was one of the fastest-growing cities in the United States when they arrived. Despite the great fire of 1871 and the economic depression that affected the entire country from 1873 to 1878, Chicago doubled in size from 1880 to 1890. With a population of nearly a million people, it was the second-largest city, behind New York, when the Rochester women arrived for school.[44]

Two years later, Edith graduated, but Dinah had contracted pneumonia while she was in school and had taken time off from her studies to recover. She graduated a year later and also returned to Rochester. Edith was originally hired by Dr. Mayo to administer anesthesia in his practice. Up until then male interns administered the chloroform, but often they became so engaged watching the operation that they neglected the patient. Dr. Mayo taught Edith to give the chloroform and monitor the patient's condition during operations conducted at his office or sometimes in a patient's home.

Dr. Mayo was by now nearing the end of his career. He was seventy years old when the hospital opened—and yet the rest of his medical team was quite young: Dr. Will was twenty-seven, Dr. Charlie twenty-three, and Edith twenty-two. Dr. Mayo found himself spending quite a bit of time convincing patients that they were in good hands despite his colleagues' youthful appearance.[45]

Since surgery was conducted only a few mornings a week, Edith worked in the Mayos' office helping with patient visits. Occasionally she had the opportunity to put her passion for swiftly riding horses to good use when Dr. Mayo urgently sent her to check on the status of a patient living in the country. She also utilized her education as the only formally trained nurse in the practice to teach the sisters assigned to Saint Marys Hospital.

In fact, Sister Joseph was one of Edith's first students shortly after she was reassigned to the hospital from her school administration position. Initially, the training did not go smoothly. One of Sister Joseph's first encounters with a patient involved a man whose body needed to be completely uncovered for examination. While the doctors and Edith completed the exam, Sister Joseph

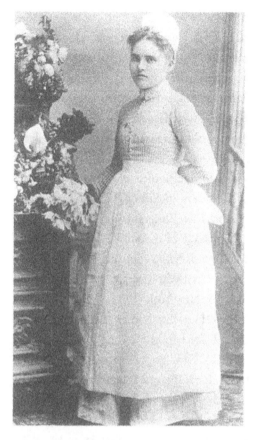

Edith Graham (Mayo)
as young nurse

turned and faced the corner in embarrassment. Afterward, she
told Miss Graham she would never be able to do this sort of work
and she intended to ask to be sent back to teach. She was convinced to stay and soon realized the importance of the nursing
tasks outweighed issues of modesty.[46]

For Sister Joseph, Rochester and Saint Marys was another adven-
ture in a circuitous life. Born Julia Dempsey on May 14, 1856, in
Salamanca, New York, to Patrick and Mary Sullivan Dempsey, she
was part of a family who had emigrated from Ireland in the 1840s
and 1850s to escape famine, poor economic conditions, and religious persecution of Catholics under the rule of Oliver Cromwell.

The conditions in Ireland were even worse than those the Moes sisters had left in Luxembourg. In Ireland, over one million people starved and two million left on "coffin ships" filled with people already too weak and ill to survive the voyage to the United States.

Patrick and Mary Dempsey made the journey in 1854 and settled in New York for ten years. Patrick worked on the railroad, and Mary maintained their household and cared for their five children, including Julia, the second oldest. Their Catholic faith was important to the Dempseys, and their decision to relocate to Minnesota was influenced by Catholic leaders, including Father John Ireland, who organized the Minnesota Irish Emigrant Society in 1864. Urging by church leaders and passage of the Homestead Act of 1862 eventually convinced the Dempseys to join relatives living near Rochester. In 1864, while the Civil War was raging in the southern states, the Dempsey family left New York.

Utilizing railroad connections that had expanded since 1851, when the Moes sisters made the trip, it took the family only ten days to journey from Buffalo, New York, to Rochester, Minnesota. They went by rail to Galena, Illinois, took a steamboat to La Crosse, Wisconsin, and rode in a covered wagon to Rochester, which at the time had a population of three thousand and was home to two newspapers, eight hotels, two breweries, seven saloons, and several churches. The Dempseys settled east of town, in Haverhill Township, along a section known as Irish Ridge. The families already established there helped the Dempseys plant their first wheat crop, which prospered.[47]

Julia, at age twenty-two, and her sister Mary were among the first postulants to join the Sisters of Saint Francis in August 1878 under Mother Alfred's leadership. They were given the names Sister Joseph and Sister Passion. Later, their younger sister Helen entered and was given the name Sister Beatrice. When the Dempseys' fourth daughter, Anna, joined the congregation, their father protested. Patrick went to the convent and took a seat in the parlor, refusing to leave until he saw Mother Alfred. When she came, he told her Anna must return home to help her mother. All of the household work now fell to her, and it was too much. Anna went home that day.[48]

In August 1890, with the capable Sister Joseph orienting to her new role in medicine, Mother Alfred finally wound down her career. After decades of nonstop work, she stepped down as administrator. Sister Hyacinth retained the role until Sister Joseph was ready to assume leadership of the hospital. Mother Alfred retired from all congregational responsibilities and moved to St. Adalbert's parish in St. Paul, living in the convent there. She helped that congregation by substitute teaching when they needed her, and she spent time in church praying.

In 1894, she moved to Sacred Heart Institute in Ironton, Ohio, where her blood sister, Sister Barbara, had been the superior since 1888. Mother Alfred enjoyed working in the garden, growing food for the congregation and visitors.

Soon Sister Barbara's health began to decline, and she died on November 23, 1895. Mother Alfred accompanied her sister's body back to Rochester for burial. When she returned to Sacred Heart Institute, she assumed her sister's position as mother superior until 1898, when, at the age of seventy, she moved to Minnesota to join her dear friend Sister Stanislaus Kostka at St. Casmir's convent in St. Paul. She also had several opportunities to visit the Franciscan congregation that she founded in Joliet, which began to celebrate her influence after resolving the severance that had occurred years earlier. And she enjoyed visiting one of the congregation's mission houses in Bayfield, Wisconsin, where they ran a school for girls near the Red Cliff Indian Reservation. This is probably as close as she came to one of her original motivations for resettling in the United States, to teach and minister among Native Americans.[49]

Toward the end of 1899, Mother Alfred grew ill and stopped traveling, despite continued invitations from the Joliet sisters and

others. When her illness became severe, Sister Sienna Otto from
Saint Marys Hospital went to St. Paul to care for her. Although
Mother Alfred initially resisted surgery, the pain of her condition
eventually drove her to accept admittance to St. Joseph's Hospital in St. Paul. She had surgery on the evening of December 17,
for what might have been a strangulated hernia. The next day, in
the company of Sisters Sienna, Kostka, and Hyacinth and Mother
Augustine, Mother Alfred died. They accompanied her body back
to Rochester by train.[50]

All charter members of the congregation were given permission to return to Rochester for services, and some came from
long distances to do so. The Bishop of Winona presided over
the funeral service, and ten priests participated. A Rochester
newspaper reported the scene in the Saint Marys chapel, where
Mother Alfred's body lay in a somber black casket, bearing a silver
plate engraved with "Mother": "It is the face of a woman whose
long life knew no idleness, a woman whose unceasing labors have
given the world monuments that will forever keep her memory
green in the hearts of suffering humanity."[51]

At seventy-one years of age, Mother Alfred was put to rest
next to Sister Barbara in St. John's Cemetery, later named Calvary
Cemetery, in Rochester, not far across town from what would
become the internationally renowned medical center she was instrumental in founding. Although the Moes sisters' forty-eight-
year journey in the United States had come to an end, their legacy
had just begun.

At the time of Mother Alfred's death, Sister Joseph had been administrator of Saint Marys Hospital for seven years. In early 1891,
she and Sister Constantine Koupal visited hospitals in St. Paul,
Minneapolis, and St. Joseph, Minnesota, as well as in Chicago to
learn about best practices at other respected facilities. In 1892, Sister
Joseph began her appointment as administrator of Saint Marys.[52]

In addition to her duties at the hospital and as religious leader for the sisters assigned there, Sister Joseph became Dr. Will's first assistant in surgery. By the end of 1893, after only three years, three thousand patients had received care at Saint Marys. Sister Joseph also led the hospital in expansions in 1894 and 1898, bringing the hospital's capacity up to 134 from its original twenty-seven beds.[53]

There was turnover among other staff, too. Charlie Mayo and Edith Graham began enjoying each other's company outside of work. Charlie was an avid bicyclist, and soon the pair was seen riding together in their time off. With their friends, they went on picnics and hayrides, and in the winter, they went ice-skating. When he traveled, Charlie wrote friendly but somewhat awkward letters to Edith. In February 1893, they went to a church supper where the cook had baked a ring in the cake; whoever found it was to receive a big blessing. No one claimed to have found the ring. They even checked in Charlie's mouth. He had cleverly hidden it, and later that evening he used the pretend ring to propose to Edith. He also gave her a copy of poetry by Ella Wheeler Wilcox. Edith accepted Charlie's proposal, and they were married on April 5 in her parent's parlor. Edith's dear friend and fellow nursing student Alice Magaw was her bridesmaid, and Charlie chose Edith's brother Dr. Christopher "Kit" Graham to be his best man, as Will was away on a trip viewing operations. Daisy Berkman, Trude's fifteen-year-old daughter and Charlie's niece, played the piano.

Charlie and Edith's honeymoon illustrated a new phase in their personal and professional partnership: they spent seven weeks visiting hospitals in New York and Chicago. Back home in Rochester, Edith's role at the Mayo practice changed. Although she would remain instrumental to the practice, she resigned her position as a nurse. Her friend and colleague Alice Magaw replaced her as anesthetist in the operating room.[54]

Edith became good friends with her sister-in-law, Hattie Damon, who had married Will Mayo nine years earlier on November 29, 1884, when Will was twenty-three and Hattie twenty. She was the only surviving child of Eleazer and Carolyn Warner Damon, originally of Massachusetts. Like Edith's parents, the Damons were among Rochester's earliest residents, having arrived in 1856 after living in Toledo, Ohio. Eleazer was a watchmaker and jeweler. The Damons opened a shop in a log frame building on what was eventually called First Avenue and later became the location of Holland's Restaurant. The Damons moved the business once more when they built a two-story brick building on Broadway, where they remained in business until retiring in 1892. The Damons' first child, Emma, died at the age of nine when Hattie was very young. Hattie went on to attend the Rochester public schools, the Rochester English and Classical School, and Carleton College. She and Will were married in her parents' home.

The following spring, Phoebe, Will and Charlie's sister, became more ill from the buggy fall she had endured seven years earlier. As a practicing physician, Will was distraught that he could not relieve his sister from the painful affliction that resisted known treatments. She died on May 15, 1885, at age twenty-eight, of an injury to the spleen, a condition Will would learn to treat—but not in time to save Phoebe's life.[55]

Two years later, Will and Hattie welcomed their first child, Carrie Louise. Their next three children, Worrall, Helen, and William Damon, born in 1889, 1892, and 1893, did not survive their first years of life. Perhaps the losses brought Will and Hattie closer. At some point in their fifty-five-year marriage, Will began calling Hattie his guiding star. In 1897, Hattie gave birth to a girl they named Phoebe Gertrude, after Will and Charlie's beloved sisters. Carrie and Phoebe would be Hattie and Will's only surviving children.[56]

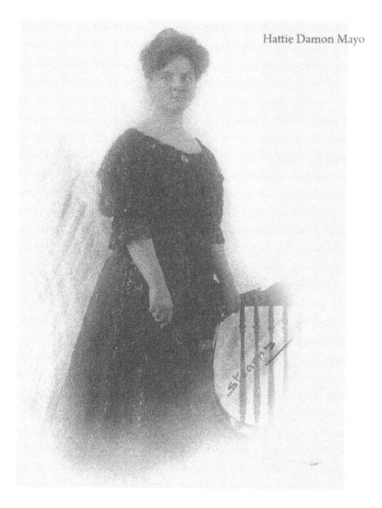

Hattie Damon Mayo

Out of the destruction of the cyclone—fallen buildings and trees, deaths and life-altering injuries—Rochester recovered, a resilient prairie town with a promising hospital and growing medical practice in its midst. Mother Alfred and Dr. William Worrall Mayo formed an unlikely collaboration, which nurtured their mutual interests: caring for humanity and reducing suffering. They began their endeavor rather late in their lives, but they skillfully mentored younger talent, men and woman who could realize their vision, perhaps beyond their most optimistic dreams.

BUILDING THE PRACTICE

1898–1906

After Saint Marys Hospital opened and was staffed by six Sisters of Saint Francis and Edith Graham, a formally educated nurse, the Mayo doctors began bringing other physicians into the practice. The third physician they added was a woman. Prior to inviting her to join them, they had collaborated with numerous women physicians who were practicing locally. Although the Mayos did not hesitate to recognize and work with women physicians, women pursuing careers in medicine encountered fierce resistance in colleges and universities and local, state, and national medical societies. Persistent, these early women physicians and nurses made significant contributions to the Mayo practice and elsewhere.

In 1898, after practicing for six months near her home, a few miles east of Rochester in the rural communities of Dover and Eyota, Dr. Gertrude Booker was invited to join the Mayo practice. She followed Edith Graham's brother, Dr. Christopher "Kit" Graham, and Dr. Augustus Stinchfield, who had established a large, successful practice in the Dover-Eyota area before joining the Mayo brothers. Dr. Stinchfield may have been the one who encouraged Gertrude to go into medicine.[1]

Born in 1871, Gertrude lived on a farm with her parents and three brothers. After her parents died when she was still a teenager, she finished high school in nearby Winona. She attended nursing school in Minneapolis, graduating in the first class of nurses at Ashbury Hospital. She then enrolled in the University of Minnesota Medical School, graduating in 1897, one of six women in a class of fifty-five. The University of Minnesota Medical School had admitted women since its opening in 1888.[2]

Dr. Booker began seeing patients at the Mayo offices in the Ramsey Building in downtown Rochester on January 1, 1898, the beginning of a tumultuous year for the United States. Cuba, one of Spain's colonies, was fighting for independence. Tensions increased, and the ten-week conflict known as the Spanish-American War resulted in the U.S. acquisition of Guam, Panama, and Puerto Rico, leaving Cuba independent. During the conflict, Annie Oakley from Ohio wrote to President McKinley, offering the government the "services of a company of 50 lady 'sharpshooters' who would provide their own arms and ammunition should war break out in Spain," evidence that women were prepared to assume roles beyond marriage and motherhood.

Around this same time, the population of Rochester reached six thousand. Communication improved with the installation of 165 telephones. City water and sewer were available. Education was provided through six public schools in addition to the Academy of Lourdes, which was built, owned, and operated by the Franciscan sisters. The Rochester congregation started by Mother Alfred was now 150 strong, supporting both teaching and healing missions. The city was also home to several mills, two glove manufacturers, two carriage makers, a camera factory, a tannery, and a woolen factory with one hundred workers, probably the largest employer in town. There was also an opera house, two bands, and an orchestra, as well as several churches and bars. Most people traveled by horse, but streetcars and railroad connections were expanding. Plans were underway for a public library building to house a collection of five thousand books. A Red Cross chapter had been organized to supply bandages and linens for soldiers involved in the Spanish-American War. According to the city directory, "the combined thrift, ingenuity, and persistence of all are united in one purpose, viz., the prosperity of all; which has produced these commendable results."[3]

The twenty-six-year-old Dr. Booker was employed as a clinical assistant to Dr. Charlie Mayo, who saw most of the eye, ear, nose, and throat cases. Her presence allowed him to devote more time to his growing surgical practice. She was particularly adept at doing eye refractions and soon assumed full responsibility for eye examinations and refractions, becoming the first Mayo physician to specialize.

Although Dr. Booker was the first woman physician employed by the Mayo family, she was not the first woman physician to work with them. Dr. Harriet Preston had arrived in Rochester from Pennsylvania thirty years earlier, in 1868, and established her office and residence in the home of Mrs. Bisbee, one door north of the Northwestern Wagon and Carriage Works on Broadway. She later established an office over Poole and Geisinger's Drug Store. Despite being considered a solid citizen and a respected physician, Dr. Preston could not be admitted to the state medical society because she was a woman.[4]

Dr. William Worrall Mayo and a couple of other physicians in support of Dr. Preston's membership sparked a discussion at the Minnesota Medical Society meeting held June 14–15, 1870, in Winona. The debate among the twenty-two physicians in attendance revealed the divided attitudes toward women in the profession.

Members in support of women argued that all qualified and recognized graduates of medicine should be included in society activities. Dr. Mayo stated that Dr. Preston was "a thoroughly competent and qualified practitioner." He was familiar with a male professor at Woman's Medical College of Pennsylvania, where she graduated, who also vouched for her competency. Further, Dr. Mayo said he met with her in consultation often and had "the highest opinion of her ability."[5]

Other physicians argued vehemently against admitting Dr. Preston. One claimed that "respect for female delicacy" would prevent him from discussing subjects like congenital malformation of a penis, a case that was on the agenda. They also noted that there was the question of physiological disability as the "only true ground upon which women can be rejected from a calling which the good sense of the mass of mankind still teaches them to believe her to be unfitted for." The membership acknowledged that the "female-woman question" was "looming up" and could not be ignored much longer. They tabled the motion, pending the credentials committee review of the situation.

At the next meeting of the society, held in St. Paul on February 8–9, 1871, with fifty-four members present, Dr. Preston's name was among a list of twenty-four physicians submitted by the credentials committee as "duly qualified for membership." Dr. Hewitt, from Red Wing, moved that "the name of Miss Preston be omitted" until action regarding the status of her alma mater was taken at the American Medical Association.[6]

The following day, the *St. Paul Weekly Press* published a record of the meeting and included the discussion about Dr. Preston's membership under the headline "No Women Need Apply." In response, the society attempted to clarify its position:

> Miss Preston's application for membership was not rejected, but merely laid over, awaiting action of the American Medical Association . . . in regard to the status of the college of which Miss Preston is a graduate. If the American Medical Association receives the Female Medical College of Philadelphia in good and regular standing with those it has already acknowledged, then Miss Preston's application can be called up and passed upon without

further debate. Her sex was not taken into consideration either by the committee or the society. But as we are governed in a great measure by the actions of the American Medical Association, we cannot accept the credentials of a graduate of a college, the position of which, in the profession, has not been passed upon by said Association.[7]

The fate of Dr. Preston's membership was sealed for a decade at the twenty-second-annual meeting of the American Medical Association held in San Francisco in May 1871. A resolution was proposed at the meeting to amend the AMA's constitution to allow delegates from female colleges. The physician who moved approval noted that the vexatious question had been before the association repeatedly and it was time to settle it. He saw no good reason why women should be prevented from practicing as physicians. He added, "They have arrived at a point when their professional ability and zeal cannot be ignored.... These women have combated against all opposition; have overcome nearly every obstacle thrown in their path, and now simply ask recognition from us—a mere recognition of them as physicians and not interlopers ... [giving] them the cold shoulder ... would be entirely inconsistent with the profession in the estimation of intelligent, right-minded people." Referring to yet another controversial topic, he also argued that not admitting women would cause them to join forces with homeopaths, which would endanger the legitimate practice of medicine.[8]

The opposition was resounding. One physician from Illinois argued that he was not comparing the relative merits of the sexes, but

Let the female remain in her sphere, and I will remain in mine.... I will say to her, "You no more can do the work designed for me than I can do the work designed for you." Woman has her sphere; man has his sphere; and the assumption that woman rises when she unsexes herself I claim to be erroneous. . . . The Creator has given the sexes distinctive features, and intended for us different spheres. The fact is unmistakable. Woman, pure woman, may be a power in the land—in her sphere. Then let her not mistake her sacred mission as wife and mother, as the light of the household.[9]

The discussion became more heated as a physician from Pennsylvania who supported the amendment was met with hisses when he claimed, "It is beneath the dignity of an association of learned scientific men to war with women." He added, if those opposed to including women "must exercise their bellicose propensities, they should enlist under General Crook, to fight the Apaches," bringing up another controversy of the time. Further, he asked the previous speaker for a definition of the woman's sphere. Did he suggest adopting India's standard "where the women were treated as brute animals"? The proponent said he had examined the records of the Female College of Philadelphia and knew that the graduates were skillful practitioners. He told the assembly that if the amendment did not pass, not only would women be precluded from membership, but members would be precluded from consulting with them according to the AMA's code of ethics.

One physician claimed that the "two sexes operating at the same dissecting table was revolting," a statement that was met with applause. Another suggested that women have an association of their own. At the end of the discussion, the subject was indefinitely postponed.[10]

The opposition to women physicians expressed at the AMA meeting represented manifestations of widespread attitudes. Women of the period were expected to stay in the home because they were considered "guardians of society and the repository of virtue." The home was deemed a safe place where they were protected from immoralities. Further, some fully believed that women were not intellectually equal to men and that they were prone to hysteria. Others felt that training women in medicine was a waste because they would all stop practicing when they married. In fact, a third of all women practitioners were married by 1900. Some never married, and some became physicians after being widowed. Others argued that even if some women stopped practicing after they married, the training was not wasted. Married women could apply what they learned in their homes and communities for the betterment of all.[11]

The AMA's and the Minnesota Medical Society's positions did not deter Dr. Mayo from praising Dr. Preston. At the conclusion of reporting a rectocele case to the membership later in 1871, Dr. Mayo noted, "I wish to make a public acknowledgement to Miss Harriet Preston, M.D., a graduate of Women's Medical College of Philadelphia, for her very able assistance to me while performing this and other operations on women such as artificial perineums, and in amputation of the cervix uteri." Publicly disclosing that he was still working with Dr. Preston after the AMA meeting could have put his membership at risk, since the AMA code did not allow for consultation outside the membership.[12]

Dr. Preston had built a successful and large practice in Rochester with a focus on gynecology and obstetrics. Many women preferred to go to a woman physician, and male practitioners were often less than adept at pelvic examinations since many of them had been trained to look at the ceiling while examining women. In addition to assisting Dr. Mayo in surgical cases, Dr. Preston referred patients to him, contributing to his growing surgical practice.[13]

Finally, in 1880, nearly a decade after Dr. Mayo's initial appeal, Dr. Preston and three other women were unceremoniously granted AMA membership. By that time, she had relocated to St. Paul, where she remained in practice until 1888, when she returned to Pennsylvania. She published and spoke on medical topics frequently, including publication in the *Northwestern Medical and Surgical Journal,* the official publication of the Minnesota Medical Society. In one article she argued that "We need more writers, more skilled physicians who can and will, like Oliver Wendell Holmes, give to the world medical facts and philosophy, in a form that will please the taste and instruct the understanding."[14]

Dr. Ida Clarke was another of the earliest physicians in Rochester to collaborate with the Mayos. She arrived in town in 1881 from Lisbon, Ohio, where she had been practicing subsequent to her graduation from the Woman's Medical College of Pennsylvania in 1878. She joined Dr. Mary Jackson Whitney in a practice specializing in obstetrics and diseases of women and children in Rochester until Dr. Whitney moved to St. Paul in 1882.

Dr. Clarke is mentioned in Rochester newspapers, which noted operations she performed or assisted with between 1881 and 1889. She frequently worked with Dr. William Worrall Mayo and Dr. Will Mayo during this period. In May 1889, she settled once again in her hometown, Youngstown, Ohio, living with her widowed mother, but she returned to Rochester and Minneapolis occasionally to visit friends. She practiced medicine in Youngstown for thirty-two years.[15]

After 1880, when women were finally admitted to the AMA and state medical societies, a period of golden opportunity arose for women in medicine. Gertrude Booker was fortunate that the doors had opened more easily for her after women like Dr. Preston and Dr. Clarke had pressed their way through. The University of Minnesota accepted men and women of all races from its beginning, in 1888. The doors did not stay open at many institutions for long, though. From the late 1800s through the turn of the century, increasing numbers of students chose to go into medicine, and a surplus of doctors began to emerge. Further, despite the AMA's efforts, the quality of physicians and their training varied greatly. Eventually, private foundations supported initiatives to improve medical education. Most notably, the Carnegie Foundation sponsored a study of medical schools conducted by Abraham Flexner. The study, known as the Flexner Report and published in 1910, established standards for faculty and facilities. Every medical school reviewed received some criticism except for Johns Hopkins University.[16]

The dictates of the Flexner Report yielded varying results. Some medical schools had to close because they were unable to meet the new standards. The report also decreased the number of medical graduates, an outcome desired by those already in the profession. By 1920, only 85 out of the 155 schools included in the report were still operating. Flexner's recommendations included that medical schools, rather than being stand-alone facilities, associate with universities that could support comprehensive academic programs; increase full-time faculty; assure rigorous coursework equating to a PhD; and enhance laboratory facilities. Significant philanthropic funding was required to make these changes at most schools.[17]

Among the hardest hit were the women's colleges because they did not have the funding that the larger private colleges and universities had. Many had to close or merge with other colleges, typically coed. The Woman's Hospital Medical College of Chicago, which received a reasonable rating in the Flexner Report, had already become the Northwestern University Women's Medical College by the time the report was published. Other schools previously for men were only beginning to open their doors to women, but women were not admitted at the same rates. Even when admitted to coed schools, women often did not feel welcome, and there were very few women on the coeducational medical school faculties, thus reducing opportunities for mentorship. Some schools, including Cornell, admitted to adopting practices intended to discourage women.[18]

The impact on the numbers of women pursuing a medical education was profound. From 1899 to 1905, women as a percentage of total enrollments dropped from 5 percent to 3.5 percent, and they dropped further in 1910, to 2.9 percent. By 1913, only 526 women were admitted to medical schools nationwide. The percentage did not rise until the 1970s, after a class action by the Women's Equity Action League against medical schools in the nation brought the "full force" of the government to bear on the discrimination. One analyst claimed, "only South Vietnam, Madagascar, and Spain have proportionately fewer women in medicine."[19]

In addition to the barriers encountered in medical schools, other factors may have accounted for the low rate of women physicians. Nursing was evolving as a profession and may have appealed to some women who might otherwise have pursued a medical degree. The field of medicine was also becoming specialized at the turn of the century, which may have deterred women who preferred more holistic approaches to caring for patients. In addition, physicians were moving away from treating patients in their homes, instead practicing in the more remote, sterile hospital environment, which may have been less appealing to some women. Opportunities in new fields, such as social work, were emerging as well.[20]

Two years after joining the Mayo practice, on Valentine's Day 1900, Dr. Booker married George W. Granger, an attorney in Rochester and later a judge. A small gathering of family and some friends, including the Stinchfields, Dr. Charlie and Edith, Trude Mayo Berkman, and her daughter Daisy, assembled for the wedding. The newspaper notice of the event stated that Dr. Booker Granger was valued at the Mayo practice and "especially capable in her chosen profession." In addition, she was "a charming lady and a social favorite." The article speculated that although she had not severed her connection with the Drs. Mayo, "it is probable that as soon as her successor can be secured, she will leave the practice of her profession for that of a homemaker." The forecast was inaccurate: Dr. Booker Granger remained in practice for nearly two decades, as long as her health allowed.[21]

George Granger's first wife had died in childbirth. His daughter, Ophelia, was two years old when he and Gertrude married. His brother's family raised the little girl. The Granger brothers and their families lived a block apart in southwest Rochester, allowing George and Gertrude to remain involved in Ophelia's life despite their busy professional obligations.

Later in 1900, on Thanksgiving Day, the Mayo practice moved from cramped quarters in the Ramsey Building across the street into new offices on the first floor of the Masonic Temple building. Dr. Booker Granger and Dr. Charlie shared an office just to the left of the entrance. Their office was quite long, about twenty feet, allowing them to conduct eye refractions.

Dr. Booker Granger's practice was busy, not only with standard exams and refractions for people needing glasses but also with complex cases. A paper she delivered in 1912 at the Olmsted Medical Society and also saw published in the medical journal *Lancet* reported on 13,000 refractions. Her paper reveals that she dealt with patients presenting a wide range of conditions: inherited retinitis pigmentosa, which frequently results in blindness; congenital cataracts, which rendered children almost visionless; detached retinas; severely injured eyes; blurred vision due to lues, the term for syphilis at the time; and toxic ambloypia believed to be caused by chemical exposure or poor nutrition. She also worked with patients who had complicated medical conditions such as sinus problems and migraines, as well as patients whose vision had been affected by a major surgery.[22]

The new space also held offices for Drs. Will Mayo, Stinchfield, Graham, and Melvin C. Millet. The frescoed walls and hardwood floors presented a pleasing appearance throughout, including in the library and reception area for visiting physicians. An x-ray

Dr. Gertrude Booker
Granger

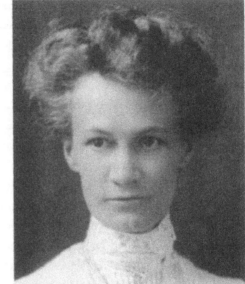

room opened into a corridor that separated the Mayo offices from the Weber & Heintz Drug Store, which occupied the other half of the first floor. A sleeping room was provided for Jay Neville, the usher, who handled maintenance among other responsibilities. The small laboratory was on the second floor. There was also an office for Alice Magaw, who provided Dr. Will with secretarial support in addition to her responsibilities anesthetizing surgical patients at Saint Marys Hospital.[23]

The Mayos had hired Alice Magaw, Edith's dear friend—maid of honor at her wedding and a fellow nursing student in Chicago—to replace Edith in administering anesthesia after she married Dr. Charlie in 1893. It was the beginning of a prolific and illustrious career that would set high standards for anesthesia administration internationally.

Alice's family moved to Rochester from Michigan in 1882, when she was twenty-two years old. Her father, a grocer, opened a store near a place in Rochester known as Five Corners. Alice became friends with Edith Graham, who was six years younger. In 1887, they enrolled in nursing school at the Women's Hospital of Chicago, and they graduated together in 1889.[24]

Alice built on what Edith had started in the operating rooms at Saint Marys Hospital. A few months into her tenure, the Mayos sent her to Chicago to study the use of a microscope for pathological specimens, and they acquired a Leitz microscope from Berlin with a magnifying power of 12,000 diameters for her to review specimens. Alice also assisted them in their offices. She handled Dr. Will's correspondence, writing letters on his behalf longhand.[25]

Alice's work anesthetizing was broadly recognized. She adopted the open drop method of slowly administering ether and chloroform, which the Mayos recently had learned from Dr. James Moore of Minneapolis, who had studied the protocol in Berlin.[26]

In 1899, Alice shared this expertise with the Olmsted Medical Society. Since she was not a physician, she was not a member of any medical society, but this invitation led to the publication of her talk in the *Northwestern Lancet*. She described her approach of talking with the patient through the process. Other methods practiced elsewhere involved "choking and smothering" the patient until the medication took effect, a "violent and dangerous practice [which] was frightening to patients and a cause of anesthetic morbidity and mortality." In contrast, Alice verbally assured the patient and slowly administered ether. A visiting surgeon noted her ability to calmly talk patients to sleep. She documented in her lectures and articles the need to carefully monitor the patient's pulse, respiration, and skin color, which she did without any of the computerized assistance now standard in surgical suites.[27]

By 1906, Alice had administered anesthesia for over 14,000 cases—more than anyone in the world had documented previously—and without an anesthesia-related death. An Iowa newspaper reported that "her remarkable work . . . has won recognition from medical authorities all over the world." Her leadership in the new field of anesthesia was such that "her work drew

Alice Magaw

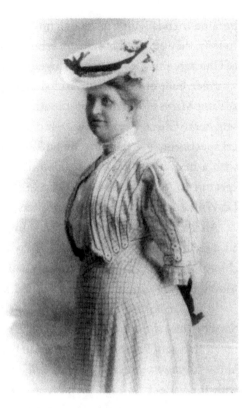

more widespread attention than that of any other member of the Rochester group apart from the Mayo Brothers themselves." In addition to traveling throughout the United States and making several trips to Europe for personal and professional purposes, she also accompanied Dr. Will and Dr. Charlie to medical meetings.[28]

Not long after Alice took over for Edith, a second full-time anesthetizer was necessary to cover the increasing surgical volume at Saint Marys Hospital. Dr. Isabella Herb of Chicago was recommended to the Mayos by a respected colleague there, and she arrived in November 1899. Dr. Herb was a graduate of the Northwestern University Women's Medical School, the renamed Women's Medical College of Chicago after its merger with Northwestern. In addition to being Dr. Charlie's anesthetist, Dr. Herb was charged with organizing the pathology department. Up until this time, the physicians, including Drs. Stinchfield and Graham, did their own laboratory work. As the number of patients increased, it seemed best to have a centralized laboratory, and Dr. Herb was hired to develop it.[29]

Dr. Herb's route to the Mayo practice and into medicine was unusual. Born Isabella Coler, she was raised in Clyman, Wisconsin. After high school, she married Charles Albert Herb, a musician from Houston, Texas, who led the twenty-four-member "Herb's Light Guard Band." Isabella lived with her husband for a few short years before he died in 1888 at age thirty-five. He and his band were performing on a barge when a bridge above them collapsed and fractured his spine. Isabella returned to Clyman for a brief period before entering medical school. She graduated in 1892, when she was about thirty years old. She completed a one-year internship at Mary Thompson Hospital for Women and Children in Chicago, where she became assistant to the medical staff and dispensary physician. She spent the next three years as an anesthetist and pathologist at Augustana Hospital in Chicago. During her tenure there, she collaborated with three other physicians studying and publishing articles on topics related to general anesthesia. Dr. Albert J. Ochsner, head of staff at Augustana Hospital, recommended Dr. Herb to the Mayos.[30]

In 1900, Dr. Herb and two local women, Daisy and Helen Berkman, began working with the Mayos. The Berkman sisters were granddaughters of Louise and William Worrall Mayo, nieces of Drs. Will and Charlie. Their mother, Trude Mayo Berkman, was busy caring for the older Mayo couple at their farm, where she moved with her family when her elderly parents needed help. Daisy, Helen, and their siblings spent some of their childhood on the farm, including time with their grandparents. Daisy loved the arts and music. She took music lessons and was known to play at family weddings. She provided the music when Edith and Dr. Charlie were married. She studied piano in Chicago and taught music lessons in Rochester before working with her uncles in their medical practice.

Daisy and Helen processed blood, sputum, and urine samples that the doctors brought back from Saint Marys Hospital and from patients examined in the downtown office. Daisy and Helen periodically ran downstairs and collected the samples for processing in the small lab on the second floor. The little room had a bench and two microscopes. When Dr. Herb arrived, she reviewed tissue samples. She worked as an anesthetist and pathologist at Saint Marys Hospital as well as in the downtown lab. Daisy also typed papers and letters for the doctors. Dr. Will was especially known for giving Daisy a handwritten draft of a paper he was going to read somewhere in the early afternoon. She typed it up, and he inevitably revised it. They went through drafts until he was happy with it. She then typed three copies: one for him to take on the four o'clock train to the meeting, one to be stored in the safe, and one mailed to arrive at the meeting.[31]

Dr. Herb and Dr. Henry Plummer, who joined the practice in 1901, did not always agree on the laboratory procedures, especially when it came to processing blood specimens. They could be heard having terrific quarrels. Other than Dr. Plummer, for these first few years, the laboratory work for the Mayo practice was conducted by four women: Dr. Herb, Alice Magaw, and Daisy and Helen Berkman.[32]

In 1904, when Dr. Herb was forty years old, she left to study in Europe for a year. She returned to the pathology laboratory at Presbyterian Hospital and Rush Medical College in Chicago, where she practiced and did bacteriology research funded by an American Medical Association grant. In 1909, she was appointed chief anesthetist at the two facilities. She published over thirty articles on pathology and anesthesiology from 1905 to 1928 as sole author. In these publications, she documented the results of her

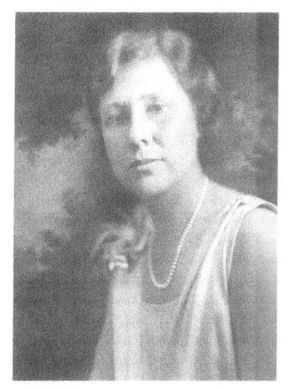

Daisy Berkman
Plummer

research, topics of clinical importance and education, including the proper roles of physicians and nurses in anesthesia administration, and the importance of anesthesia education for medical students and interns. In 1916, she became the tenth president of the American Association of Anesthetists and was given an award for "meritorious services in the art and teaching of anesthesia."

Dr. Herb retired in 1941 as professor of surgery (anesthesia) after teaching hundreds of students and "several score" of interns. Although her ambition had been to become a surgeon, she finished a distinguished career working alongside many preeminent surgeons as an anesthetist for forty-three years. She died two years later, on May 28, 1943, and was buried in Clyman, Wisconsin, her hometown.[33]

Dr. Herb was not the only one of the three women working in the laboratory to leave in 1904. One day when Dr. Plummer and Daisy were working together, he turned to shut off a water faucet and casually said, "Daisy Berkman, I'd like to marry you." Daisy did not immediately take him up on the suggestion. A courtship began. Henry wrote to her whenever he traveled to other medical centers and medical meetings. Despite his reputation for being fervently dedicated to his work, his love for her was revealed in stacks of letters that she kept.[34]

Eventually, Henry convinced Daisy, and they were married on October 6, 1904. Gertrude "Trude" Mayo Berkman and Dr. David M. Berkman, Daisy's parents, hosted seventy-five colleagues, family members, and friends. The bride wore a gown of crepe de Chine trimmed in Cluny lace, and she carried a bouquet of marguerites. The parlor and dining room were decorated with smilax, pink asters, and red roses. The couple left on the evening train for Chicago. Some of their honeymoon was spent shopping for furniture for their new home on West Zumbro Street, which Henry designed.[35]

Unprecedented numbers of women were involved in the Mayo practice in its very earliest years. These physicians, nurses, and laboratory technicians provided extraordinary care to patients. They would soon be joined by women in many other fields as the Mayo practice expanded.

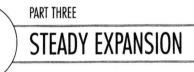

PART THREE

STEADY EXPANSION

REACHING AROUND THE GLOBE

1907–1913

The Mayo practice was no longer a doctor's office just for the people in Rochester and the surrounding areas. The Mayos and their colleagues began drawing patients from greater distances as their reputation grew. Physicians from around the country visited to see what the Mayos were doing so successfully. As the practice expanded, more women were added in a wide range of positions, clinical and administrative. But the women's contributions were not limited to the Mayo practice; they also made significant improvements in the growing community.

"We want you, we want you badly, and the sooner the better," Dr. Will Mayo wrote to Maud Mellish on January 1, 1907. "I think you will like it here. You will have a permanent position and run the library end of the business." Maud had been recommended to the Mayos by Dr. Albert J. Ochsner, a trusted friend and colleague practicing in Chicago who had also recommended Dr. Isabella Herb a few years earlier.[1]

Dr. Will's letter was followed by another on February 12, in which he displayed somewhat uncharacteristic humor in his attempt to recruit Maud: "Bring the dog, of course, everybody expects him and never had any idea to the contrary. All of the folks here keep at least one dog and most of them two. We indulge in one, but Dr. Charles has three, Dr. Millet four, Dr. Wilson five, etc.... At present, you will stay with Mrs. Mayo's mother and they need a dog so they say."[2]

At first, Maud was hesitant to move to Rochester, a prairie town of eight thousand people, after living in Chicago. Since the late 1880s, when Edith Graham had studied nursing there, Chicago had doubled in population to over two million people. Industry and the arts were flourishing in the city. It had hosted the World's Fair in 1893, the Art Institute of Chicago and the Chicago Orchestra were vibrant, and theater and opera performances abundant.[3]

Despite her reservations, Maud made a visit to Rochester and was convinced to join the Mayo practice as librarian and editor. She truly came in at the ground level; there was hardly a library to speak of. Her first order of business was to centralize the meager book collection, which consisted mostly of holdings scattered in the individual physicians' offices. Maud discovered that past issues of journals and even some manuscripts that the Mayo physicians had submitted for publication had been thrown away. She rescued some of them from the coal bin, to the amusement of the maintenance man, who had put them there.[4]

At the time of Maud's arrival, the Mayo offices were still in the Masonic Temple building in downtown Rochester. Nine physicians were affiliated with the practice, plus a staff of twenty-five nurses, laboratory technicians, and other positions. That year, 1907, saw the largest growth in the small practice to date. Nine people, including Maud, were hired, bringing the number of physicians and other staff to forty.

Initially, the library was quite small, originating in the front room of the offices and including a large window and an easy chair, often occupied by Dr. William Worrell Mayo, now eighty-seven years old. Maud had three book stacks, a reading table, and more chairs installed. She then turned her attention to expanding the collection through acquisitions and made arrangements to borrow material from the surgeon general's library and other libraries when necessary.

Maud had come full circle when she returned to Minnesota in 1907. She was born near the farming community of Faribault, sixty miles northeast of Rochester. She was the seventh and youngest child of Peter and Sarah Moses Headline. Her parents emigrated from Sweden in 1851, the same year that Mother Alfred and her sister arrived from Luxembourg and that Louise Wright married William Worrall Mayo. The family first settled in Chicago, but in 1855 after a cholera epidemic broke out and eventually claimed the lives of fourteen hundred people, they traded their modest home and property for a team of horses and a buggy and moved forty miles west to St. Charles, Illinois. Soon they continued to south central Minnesota, eventually settling on a farm near Faribault, where Annie Maud Headline was born on Valentine's Day 1862.[5]

Annie Maud was very curious as a child. She wanted to know how everything worked and the causes of things in her surroundings. She took insects apart to learn their anatomy, and she convinced her playmates to allow mosquitoes to remain on their arms and legs until the insects were filled with blood because she was convinced doing so would prevent a lump from appearing. She was always finding something that interested her.[6]

Four months a year, Annie attended a country school a mile and a half from the farm. During years when there was a lack of funding for the local school, she and her siblings walked three and a half miles to the next closest school. Annie remained enthusiastic about learning and satisfying her curiosity despite being nearly blind in one eye. Several years later, doctors determined that she had a cataract, and when it was removed in her twenties, her sight was restored. After completing her education in the public schools at age sixteen, Annie attended an academy in Medford, Minnesota, about ten miles away. Before she could finish a second year, one of her sisters became ill, and Annie stayed home to help care for her. Her sister's physician was impressed with Annie's assistance and encouraged her to pursue a medical career.

In 1885, Annie enrolled in a nurse's training course in Chicago.

She did not have the resources to support herself in medical school, so she chose the nursing program at Presbyterian Hospital because of its association with and proximity to Rush Medical College. During nursing school, she was allowed to sit in on many medical courses, and she impressed the faculty. She graduated in May 1887, the same year Edith Graham arrived at Chicago Women's Hospital to begin nursing school and Gertrude Booker graduated from the University of Minnesota Medical School. Annie worked as a private duty nurse before becoming the superintendent of the Maurice Porter Memorial Hospital for Children.[7]

On September 28, 1889, when Annie was twenty-seven years old and before her nursing career progressed very far, she married Dr. Ernest J. Mellish, a promising young surgeon. Sometime after their marriage, she began to use Maud, her middle name, instead of Annie. They moved to Ishpeming, Michigan, where her husband practiced until 1893, when they returned to Chicago. Despite the opulent celebration of the World's Fair that year, an economic panic struck the country. Railroad speculation and bank failures caused unemployment rates to reach and remain at double digits for five years. Along with the rest of the nation, the Mellishes struggled financially. Ernest practiced medicine in charity hospitals and was an instructor at Rush Medical School. Maud got her first experience editing by reviewing several of his medical articles. He noted, "Maud is of inestimable aid to me in revising my papers. I am sure they are much more readable for the revision. There are no superfluous words left in them."[8]

In addition to their financial challenges, Ernest battled tuberculosis, which he had contracted before they were married. His illness made it difficult for him to work. Fortunately, the disease went into remission in 1897, allowing him to rebuild his practice until 1901, when its recurrence led them to relocate to El Paso, Texas, where he again maintained a successful practice until ultimately the tuberculosis triumphed. Ernest died on April 23, 1905, widowing Maud after nearly sixteen years of marriage. At forty-three years old, she returned to Chicago and found work among their medical friends, organizing a library for Augustana Hospital and editing for Dr. Albert J. Ochsner. She was there when Dr. Will Mayo sent the letter requesting that she consider employment in Rochester.

In addition to making acquisitions for the library, Maud began the most enduring of her contributions to the practice soon after her arrival. Dr. Will noted that the "character of the papers contributed by the members of the staff was not up to the standard of the clinical work." The publication of papers was extremely important in extending Mayo's reputation beyond its rather remote midwestern location. A physician's standing in the medical community and, consequently, patient referrals were dependent on publishing high-quality articles about his or her practice. So, Maud applied her finely tuned editorial skills to the papers written by the physicians at Mayo.

Maud was considered a tough critic. She strove to assure accuracy and truth in an article while preserving the author's tone and voice. Her background in nursing and the medical courses she had taken in Chicago were helpful to her in the editing process and added to her credibility with the physicians.

Once, before departing on a trip, Dr. Charlie left with her a paper he had written. When he returned several weeks later, he saw an article on his desk and read it. He thought it was quite good and wondered who had written it—until he realized it was a revision of his paper, the result of Maud's editing.

Maud also taught new staff members how to research scientific articles and prepare presentations. She wrote a book, *The Writing of Medical Papers*, as a guide for physicians. Her tough approach is evident in some of the advice it included:

Don't always go back to the Garden of Eden to review the literature to date.

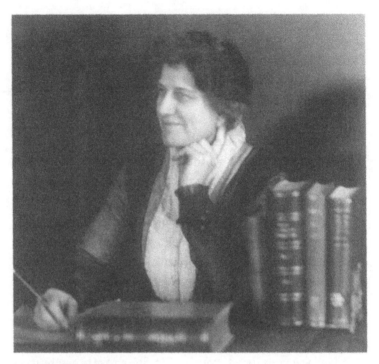

Maud Mellish Wilson

Don't estimate measurements in terms of coconuts, oranges, . . . eggs, beans and so forth; use the metric system.

Don't forget that skipping about from tense to tense in one paragraph has not even a Bergsonian justification. It is blasphemous, ungrammatical, and annoying.[9]

In addition to editing individual papers written by Mayo physicians, Maud became the impetus behind the publication of *The Collected Papers of the Mayo Clinic,* from 1909 an annual and sometimes semiannual publication that accumulated the best articles written by Mayo physicians during the year. Maud selected the articles and edited the collections. By the end of her tenure, she had chosen and edited over six thousand articles representing

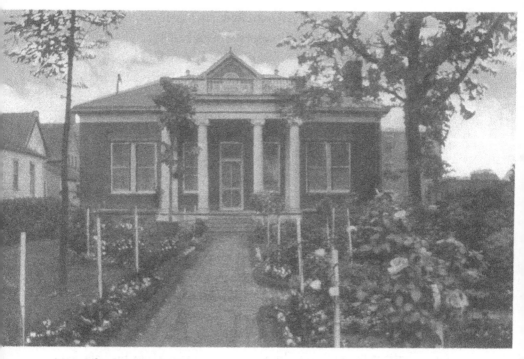

Mayo Library, 1909

the very latest medical knowledge produced by Mayo physicians. These volumes were instrumental in spreading the name of Mayo Clinic nationally and internationally beyond its rather modest and remote location in the prairies of southeastern Minnesota. During these years, medical advertising and promotion was at times illegal and nearly always considered unethical. The Mayos shunned recognition by the media, even articles by periodicals such as *Life* magazine, for fear of criticism. *The Collected Papers of the Mayo Clinic* under Maud's purview became one of the most important ways, in addition to traveling and lecturing, to spread word of the work they were doing.[10]

By 1909, the library had outgrown the front room of the offices and a small, separate structure was built on an adjacent lot and connected to the Masonic Temple building by a corridor.

The first floor contained a spacious reading room with expansive bookcases and a large circular revolving reading table and several study tables. This room was also used for staff meetings and lectures. In addition, two smaller rooms were used for editorial work and other routine library processing. The second floor contained the art studio, used to create illustrations for articles, as well as coat and storage rooms. Maud quickly began filling this building. One of the most beautiful gardens in downtown Rochester was established in its small front yard, the beginning of elegant grounds that became a part of the Mayo culture.

While Maud Mellish was busy building the library and editing papers for publication, Mabel Root was hired in 1907 to organize the patient records. Up until that time, the doctors had maintained their own individual ledgers of patient histories. This process became problematic when someone wanted to review, for example, gallbladder cases seen by all of the doctors. Also, if a patient was to be seen by a second doctor at Mayo, the "big book would need to be hauled" from one doctor to another. In addition, operations were recorded at Saint Marys Hospital and not included in the downtown records. When ancillary areas like the laboratories and radiology began generating patient test results, there was even greater need to centralize and organize all patient information into one accessible record.

Dr. Henry Plummer, who had joined the practice in 1905, conceptualized an integrated medical record that would include all aspects of a patient's medical history regardless of who in the practice provided the care. This comprehensive medical record would become a critical cornerstone in establishing the successful group practice of medicine model that was evolving among the Mayos and their associates. Mabel Root was hired to implement the system. The attention to detail she exhibited in her previous employment in Rochester at E. A. Knowlton's dry goods store was important to the success of the new system.[11]

While Dr. Plummer had a vision for how this system would work, he "was the type of man that gave each worker an opportunity to work out the details for themselves." So, Mabel Root did just that. She took the lead with new patient record forms and the six wood file cabinets that were installed in the offices at the Masonic Temple. She worked to encourage doctors to use the new system that ultimately accumulated all clinical, surgical, laboratory, and follow-up correspondence into one unified, color-coded patient record. Some physicians, such as Dr. Booker Granger, who only saw eye patients, did not initially appreciate the need for the new system, but Mabel worked to convince them. She and some of the other staff transcribed information out of the old ledger books and added the past surgical cases from Saint Marys Hospital. In the process, Mabel discovered some patients had no clinic record at all because they had been taken directly to the hospital by the doctors, whose "first care was for the patient."[12]

In addition to creating the new record system and beginning to assign each record with a unique number, there was a need to index the surgical cases and clinical diagnoses. The index would facilitate research and, ultimately, the clinic's mission of improving care. Mabel, who was a good friend of Daisy Plummer's, worked evenings at the Plummer home so Dr. Plummer could teach her how to accurately classify the medical and surgical information.

Mabel recalled those early days as "breath taking and exciting. . . . Nobody kept any regular hours. Patients began arriving at six o'clock in the morning" on the train. She and Cora Olson, among others, registered the patients. Cora also handled much of the correspondence for the physicians before secretaries were hired for each of them. At times she would be at the desk registering patients and "one of the doctors might come along and start dictating letters to her." They worked every day, including Sundays, for a long time. New Year's Day was the only day off. They worked until one in the afternoon on Christmas and other holidays.[13]

Mabel Root

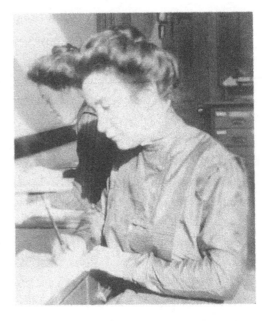

In 1908, Dr. Leda Stacy became the third woman physician brought into the Mayo practice. Three of the first fifteen physicians affiliated with the practice were women. Born in Rochester in 1882, Leda was inspired by the local homeopath, Dr. Allen, who brought little No. 1 and No. 2 bottles with him when he made house calls. When Leda expressed interest in nursing, her father suggested that she become a doctor, "as it had a greater future." She attended Rush Medical College in Chicago, graduated in 1905, and interned for a year at Children's Hospital in San Francisco, where she experienced the great earthquake that shook that city in 1906.[14]

After Dr. Stacy's return to Rochester, Dr. Will Mayo asked her if she would be interested in joining the staff as an anesthesiologist. She accepted and began at Saint Marys Hospital as Dr. E. Starr Judd's anesthetist. She learned the anesthesiology practice from Alice Magaw, who had fifteen years of experience by then. In addition to Alice Magaw, Florence Henderson and Mary Hines administered anesthesia at Saint Marys Hospital, supporting the increasingly busy surgical practice. In 1908, Dr. Will, Dr. Charlie, and two other staff surgeons and their assistants performed 6,454 surgical procedures there.[15]

Shortly after Dr. Stacy's arrival, Alice Magaw's career changed. Dr. George Kessel, a prominent surgeon and owner of Kessel Hospital in Cresco, Iowa, came to know Alice through his associations with the Mayo brothers. At six o'clock in the evening on May 23, 1908, at age forty-seven, Alice married George Kessler in Dr. Will and Hattie's home on West College Street.[16]

The bride was escorted by her brother under an arch of woven ornamental asparagus ferns and through a lane of ribbons held by the flower girls, including one of the groom's daughters. Daisy Plummer played the wedding march from *Lohengrin* during the processional. Dr. Will was best man. Thirty-eight people, primarily members of the Mayo practice and a few friends and family members, joined the couple for a candlelit dinner served in the library. After dinner, the couple left by the evening train for St. Paul and eventually Quebec, where they boarded the *Empress of Ireland* for a three-month European tour.[17]

One newspaper recognized Alice's illustrious and prolific career in the description of the wedding. Remembered as a woman of "rare virtues and sunny disposition," Alice was the only full-time anesthetizer for the Mayo practice for the first seven years of her career, and in the entire fifteen years that she worked in that capacity over 17,000 persons were "safely carried through a period of insensibility to pain."[18]

The transition from being a single professional woman to a married woman and stepmother was a big change for Alice. She continued to administer anesthesia in the Kessel and St. Joseph's Mercy Hospitals. Occasionally the Mayo brothers operated alongside her husband, so she remained in contact with them. Alice's new family included four daughters. George had been widowed, and two of the girls were still at home. Some accounts claim that the girls resisted her presence. Alice was expected to entertain and be a successful surgeon's wife and fulfill her professional role. Even though she had hired staff to help at home, she preferred to do many of the chores herself. After eleven years, on August 7, 1919, Alice and George signed a legal separation. Couples preferring not to divorce for financial or religious reasons legally separated. She was subsequently listed as Alice Magaw, widow of Kessel in the Rochester city directories.[19]

Alice returned to work at Saint Marys Hospital. By then there were several anesthetizers on staff, and Alice was not as prominent. She stopped working in 1925, when she was sixty-five years old. Her health declined and she died of complications from diabetes in 1928 after spending nearly two months in a sanitarium in Hudson, Wisconsin. She was buried with many of her family in Corunna, Michigan, the town of her childhood. Her contributions to the field were significant enough that later professionals considered her the "Mother of Anesthesia."[20]

Shortly after the library annex building was opened in 1909, Sophia Tandberg Hogenson was hired and listed in the practice's records as the first janitress. The practice now had a substantial amount of office space in the Masonic Temple in addition to this new small building. Sophia had immigrated to the United States from Norway in 1869 when she was ten years old. Her parents settled in Spring Grove, Minnesota, with Sophia and her five siblings. Sophia married Severt Hogenson, another Norwegian immigrant, when she was twenty-one, and they farmed nearby in Rock Dell on property owned by her husband's brother. They had four sons and three daughters.

In 1907, Sophia's husband was killed in a horse and buggy accident, leaving her to support three children still living at home, the youngest only three years old. Soon after the accident, her brother-in-law asked her to leave the farm. Sophia borrowed money from some relatives and bought a small, simple home in Rochester. She began work cleaning at the Mayo offices and library. She also

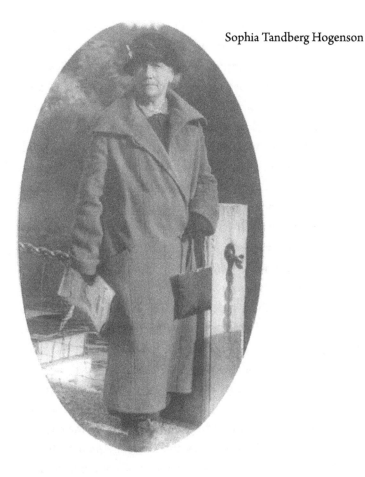

Sophia Tandberg Hogenson

picked up additional jobs doing housework for some of the doctors' families, including Dr. Will and Hattie. During her tenure, three of her adult sons died: Peter from a gas accident in 1910, George in 1918 in France during the war, and Edwin the same year of influenza. Despite these losses, Sophia persevered and encouraged her children to get good educations; many went on to professional careers in nursing and engineering. Sophia continued as the janitress for fifteen years, until she was sixty-six years old. She subsequently suffered a stroke and, tragically, was burned when a heater near her wheelchair ignited and the blanket covering her caught fire.[21]

During these early years as the staff grew, the Mayo families in-creased in number and in size as well. Most physicians invited to join the practice were married, especially the men, or they married soon. A certain sense of respectability was associated with being married at the time. With the expanding list of physicians, there were additional spouses, mostly women. In addition to their roles as wives and mothers, the women wanted to be knowl-edgeable and well read. In 1911, when there were thirty-seven phy-sicians, nearly all of them with spouses, the Magazine Club was organized. On a train ride from Minneapolis to Rochester, Helen Berkman Judd, Daisy's sister and one of the first laboratory tech-nicians prior to her marriage to Dr. E. Starr Judd, and Elizabeth Brackenridge, married to Christopher Graham, came up with the plan for the women to meet.

Helen and Elizabeth's idea was based on the Surgeons Club, which was organized among the Mayo physicians in 1906 and met every week to discuss interesting cases and the latest medical news. The members of the Magazine Club decided to meet on Monday afternoons because it was washday and almost everyone would be home and free of other commitments. They took turns hosting the meetings and reading and reporting on the contents of important magazines, such as the *Nation, Atlantic Monthly, Outlook, Century,* and *Scribner's,* as a way of staying current on national and international events. They also discussed music, the-ater, gardening, and literary works by Wordsworth, Keats, Tenny-son, and Austin.[22]

On March 6, 1911, a month after their sixtieth wedding anniver-sary, Louise Mayo's husband, Dr. William Worrall Mayo, died at ninety-one years old. Months earlier, he had been searching for a way to extract ethanol from animal and vegetable wastes for use as fuel when his hand and lower arm were crushed in a machine. Despite treatment and two operations, Dr. Mayo died of nephritis, a kidney disease related to complications from the accident and related pain. Prior to the accident, Dr. Mayo had been extraordinarily active, traveling to distant places including Mexico, China, and Japan. Although Louise stayed home while William was away, she read so extensively about the countries he visited that he referred friends to her because she could often answer their questions about his travels better than he could.[23]

Louise and William's daughter Trude Mayo Berkman and her family had been caring for her parents as they aged. Within a year of her father's death, Trude's husband, Dr. John Berkman, a retired veterinarian, died of cancer, leaving Trude a widow at fifty-eight years old. She traveled to interesting places such as Cuba to recover from the losses of her father and husband, and she continued to care for Louise. Almost all of her children were connected to the Mayo practice in some way. Her daughter Daisy was married to Dr. Plummer, and her daughter Helen was married to Dr. E. Starr Judd. Her son Dr. David Berkman joined the Mayo practice in 1913. Her other son, John, was only fourteen when his father died, but he, too, went on to become a Mayo physician.

In the fall of 1911, months after William Worrall Mayo's death, Dr. Charlie and Edith had a scare while on a trip to the East Coast for medical meetings. After spending time in Washington, DC, they were in New York City when Charlie suddenly became ill. Although he sensed he had gallstones, the New York surgeon disagreed and removed his appendix. Dr. Charlie's condition became life threatening.

When Dr. Will heard about his brother's illness, he and Dr. Charlie's anesthetist, Florence Henderson, made a record-breaking trip by train to New York, where Dr. Will operated on Charlie and removed his troublesome gallbladder. Edith and Dr. Charlie remained in New York while he regained his strength.

They returned to Rochester in January to celebrate a belated Christmas with their family, which by this time included six children, ranging in age from toddler to teen.

By the time of this near-tragic event, Edith and Charlie had been married fifteen years. They lost their first infant girl during her first year of life. Dorothy, their second child, nearly died from scarlet fever in 1900, when she was a toddler. Edith's nursing expertise probably saved Dorothy's life when she fell into a fever-induced coma, but the high temperature caused brain damage that prevented Dorothy from developing into a self-sufficient adult. Edith sometimes wondered if she had done the right thing when she saw Dorothy's discouragement with her own limitations in comparison to what her siblings were able to accomplish.[24]

These disappointments and the loss of their two-year-old baby, Rachel, in 1910 due to an intestinal disorder brought dark days, but otherwise Edith and her family lived happy, busy lives in a house next door to Dr. Will and Hattie and their two girls. Dr. Will and Dr. Charlie were often away observing medical practices or at meetings, and when they were home, their surgical practices kept them busy at the office and hospital. They conducted all of the operations, nearly three thousand a year, until 1905 when Dr. E. Starr Judd was added.[25]

After Edith and Charlie were first married in 1893, they lived with Hattie and Will in the "yellow house" on College Street for two years until they built their own, very similar house, the "red house," next door. Charlie had lived with his brother and sister-in-law in the yellow house before he married Edith.

Edith and Charlie's home was three stories high with open porches on two stories and a cupola exuding the Queen Anne Victorian style, but much of the interior was of the simpler American Arts and Crafts style. Charlie's library was the largest room in the house and had Frank Lloyd Wright–like features, including built-in bookcases, beveled glass doors, leaded and stained glass windows, and cherry and white oak interior. The home was spacious, with thirteen bedrooms and plenty of room for their family, household staff, and visiting physicians. They entertained frequently, holding dinners for fifty people and hosting a dancing club. Even after the medical practices became too busy for much socializing, they hosted friends' weddings and other special dinners. Charlie was known for inviting guests home with little notice, so Edith learned to keep a well-stocked pantry. Edith did much of the cooking herself in the early years.[26]

In addition to living next door to each other, the Mayos shared a bank account. The brothers were extremely close. They also had a double rocking chair built so they could sit together in the evening while discussing the events of the day. At one point, they suggested building a corridor between the houses with a joint study and library. Edith and Hattie vetoed the plan, deciding that the brothers had enough togetherness, and probably fearing they would see even less of their husbands than they already did.[27]

Charlie and Edith enjoyed the countryside and often took carriage rides and went picnicking. Soon, they decided to build a country place they called Ivy Cottage. One day when they were out with their children on a favorite spot among the rolling hills and along the Zumbro River, Charlie took out some string and started to mark off plans for a larger home, in part so that their children would have an opportunity to enjoy the farm life that he and Edith had known at times during their childhoods. Charlie drew the plans himself, in the Arts and Crafts style without any of the more ornate look of their first home.

Construction began in 1911 for a home with thirty-eight rooms on four floors, including a ballroom, a conservatory for stargazing inspired by Louise, and a music room. They built a dam on the river to generate electricity and form a lake. The grounds of "Mayowood" eventually included a greenhouse, eight ponds, a tempietto, a pergola, a teahouse, statues, stables, a racetrack for horses, and a garage. In 1900, Charlie had been the first person in Rochester to own a car. Over time, Edith and Charlie acquired

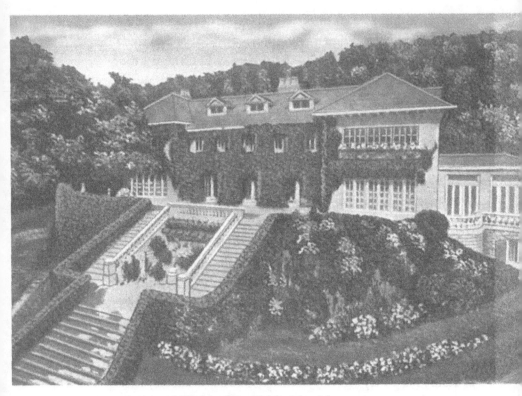

Mayowood, Edith and Dr. Charlie Mayo's home

more than three thousand acres, including eight working farms with beef and dairy cattle, hogs, and various crops. Charlie populated the grounds with exotic wildlife, including Japanese deer, bison, elk, and peacocks.[28]

The couple gave the red house to the YWCA, one of the organizations that Edith helped found. In addition to her commitment to her family and her husband's career, she was a leader in the community in various ways, including organizing the YWCA and the Civic League. The women involved in the league were truly activists, "promoting better and cleaner conditions in Rochester." Edith's sister-in-law Trude Berkman had helped organize the Rochester Women's Club, a predecessor to the Civic League. The women saw the need for many improvements in citizens' health and welfare, and they "had the courage to" implement the changes "when no other existing body was authorized to do so."[29]

The list of accomplishments for the Rochester Women's Club and its successor organization is impressive. Among their earliest accomplishments, in 1894, was establishing a public restroom for women and children, who had no place to clean up when coming to town to shop or attend to other errands. It was the first of its kind in the nation. They also established cooking classes and a free kindergarten and hired visiting nurses, a school nurse, and a health inspector. These programs were the predecessors to the public health department and the public school nurse program.

In 1912, scarlet fever reached epidemic levels and Edith's work with the Civic League converged with Charlie's work. Many citizens, including league members, were not convinced that the city's health officer was doing enough to abate the spread of the disease. Perhaps because Edith and Charlie's daughter, Dorothy, had been afflicted by it in 1900, Edith was especially passionate about the threat. Charlie was also concerned because reports of the epidemic might discourage people from coming to Rochester to seek medical care. Their efforts resulted in Charlie becoming Rochester's health officer. He immediately established strict quarantine guidelines and worked with Sister Joseph and the Sisters of Saint Francis to renovate a hotel for use as an isolation hospital.[30]

In addition to addressing the scarlet fever epidemic, the Civic League, with both Edith and Hattie involved, advocated for the first woman member on the school board, a policewoman, a truant officer, milk and meat inspections, school inspections, garbage removal, enforcement of the curfew for children under the age of sixteen, and an ordinance prohibiting spitting in public places. They helped establish a dental clinic for children, school gardens, and a weekly health lecture. Over a hundred women were involved, along with twenty men.[31]

The Mayo practice was growing at accelerating rates. In 1893, the Mayos performed just under 500 surgical procedures. Five years later, in 1898, the number doubled, bringing the total to 1,100. By 1903, the practice more than doubled again, and Dr. Will and Dr. Charlie performed 2,640 surgeries. After they added another surgeon in 1905, and another in 1908, over 6,000 surgical procedures were performed. By 1911, forty-one men and eighteen women were employed with the Mayo practice in addition to the Sisters of Saint Francis, who staffed the hospital.[32]

From the time of its opening in 1889 to 1912, Saint Marys Hospital expanded five times, resulting in the availability of nearly three hundred beds, over ten times its original count. Other facilities opened in Rochester to help meet patients' needs, including the Kahler Hospital and Chute Sanatorium, which provided another 150 beds by 1911.[33]

With the accelerating growth in patients and the related additions to the staff, the Mayos began plans to erect a building dedicated entirely to their practice. In 1912, the house where Dr. Charlie had been born and Dr. William Worrall Mayo had died was razed to make way for the first Mayo Clinic building. At the ground-breaking ceremony, Dr. Will Mayo said, "The object of this building is to furnish a permanent house wherein scientific investigation can be made into the cause of the diseases which afflict mankind, and wherein every effort shall be made to cure the sick and suffering. . . . Within its walls all classes of people, the poor as well as the rich, without regard to color or creed, shall be cared for without discrimination."[34]

THE NEEDS OF THE PATIENT COME FIRST

1914–1919

As the Mayo practice grew and evolved into a clinic dedicated to the best interests of the patient, women were involved in nearly every aspect. They led innovative clinical and research initiatives. Some of their roles—for example, as artists—were extraordinarily unique. And they applied their skills in unconventional settings outside of the clinic and Rochester, serving their country alongside some of the men during World War I.

Sixteen hundred people arrived for the opening reception and tour of the new Mayo Clinic building in downtown Rochester on Friday, March 6, 1914. The four-and-a-half-story red brick building stood on the site of the first home that Louise and William Worrall Mayo had built fifty years before when they moved to town in 1864. From five to nine o'clock in the evening, guests streamed into a lobby finished with fumed oak walls, cork floors, wicker furniture, and large palms. The room was designed to comfortably hold 350 waiting patients, but could accommodate 550 people if necessary. A large fountain in the center was surrounded with colorful potted plants. An orchestra played while women of the Civic League served refreshments. Revenue from hosting the event would provide funding for their visiting nurse program.[1]

One newspaper reported that the decorative touches, peaceful surroundings, and alluring appointments "are conducive to a forgetfulness of one's physical suffering, calling forth the higher instinct of love for the aesthetic and sublime, giving to the broken in spirit a new vision that dispels gloom and bids him who enters here not all hope to abandon."[2]

Employees, including the heads of departments, greeted visitors as they made their way through the building, designed by Dr. Plummer to facilitate an efficient flow of patients and records. One Rochester newspaper described the layout as one "which will produce the accomplishment of the greatest possible good in the smallest possible time . . . that the work may be accomplished with the highest degree of harmony and precision." A medical journal article noted that beyond the commitment of "the group of men and women who compose the Mayo Clinic" to diagnose and treat patients, the facility supported scientific investigation and educational activities instrumental to furthering the medical profession.[3]

The Mayo Clinic was considered the first structure built specifically for a private group practice of physicians, and it facilitated the holistic approach to patient care advocated by Dr. William Worrall Mayo years earlier and refined by Drs. Will and Charlie: that the patient be treated by a group of specialists who function in unison. Dr. Will told the Rush Medical College graduating class of 1910, "The best interest of the patient is the only interest to be considered, and in order that the sick may have the benefit of advancing knowledge, union of forces is necessary. . . . It has become necessary to develop medicine as a cooperative science; the clinician, the specialist, and the laboratory workers uniting for the good of the patient."[4]

Forty physicians were involved in the practice when the building opened. Quite self sufficient, the facility included maintenance shops where surgical instruments were designed and manufactured, stenographers' desks, files for patient records, and a greenhouse, where flowers were grown by a skillful gardener for the lobby and routing desks throughout the building. In addition to these support functions and the clinically focused examination

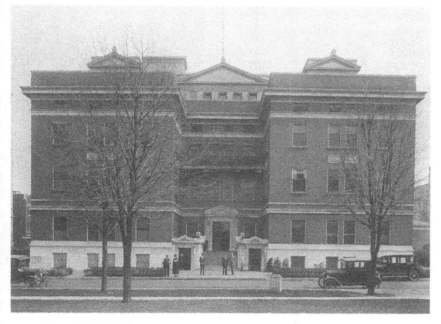

Mayo Clinic Building, 1914

rooms, procedural areas, x-ray facilities, and laboratories, Maud
Mellish's library was moved out of the annex building and into
half of the third floor of the new building. The library and editorial staff, the stacks containing four thousand volumes, reading
and smoking rooms, and an assembly room were designed to support the educational activities of the practice.[5]

In addition to overseeing the library and editing manuscripts,
Maud was also responsible for the art department. Mayo physicians began including photography and hand-drawn illustrations
in their publications in 1905. Dr. Louis Wilson, who joined the
practice that year to head the laboratory after Dr. Herb left, was
interested in photography. He worked with the medium himself,
and photographers were soon hired to capture patient conditions
and both gross and microscopic specimens. While photography
was accurate, it was not as helpful in portraying sequential steps

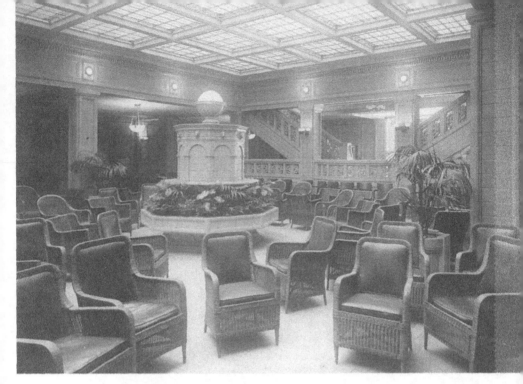

Mayo Clinic Building lobby

in surgery or illustrating potential processes. Further, all photography of the time was limited to black-and-white images. Thus, hand-drawn, sometimes color illustrations became important features in many of the papers written by Mayo physicians.[6]

Outside artists were utilized to provide illustrations until 1907, when Florence Byrnes from Boston was hired; she remained in the position until 1909, when she married. Next, a local woman, Dorothy Peters, was hired and sent to New York to study with Max Brödel, a renowned medical illustrator at Johns Hopkins University. The Mayos recognized that his "beautiful drawings . . . did much to help establish Hopkins as a leader in surgical education and research." After Dorothy Peters left the position in 1912, Eleanora Fry, a New York artist who studied at the well-known Pratt Institute, was hired. In addition to medical illustration, her work had been included in the prestigious New York Watercolor Club exhibit. Her talent was recognized in a review of a cystoscopy book published in the December 1911 issue of the *American Surgi-*

cal Journal: "The work is illuminated by numerous (233) excellent illustrations ... drawn from life by Miss Eleanor [*sic*] Fry. . . . She deserves much of the credit that will attach to this book no less as a manual of instruction than as a work of pictorial elegance."[7]

Eleanora Fry arrived in Rochester in 1912 with her parents. She was twenty-eight years old, and her mother was blind. Eleanora was the head of the art studio, even after two men were hired. Coworkers described her as a "serious, hardworking no-nonsense person whose entire life consisted of her art and her family." She had a "slow methodical way of working out a whole drawing," quietly with great solemnness and concentration. She sat still, hardly moving or speaking to others for hours until the drawing was done to her satisfaction. When new comfortable chairs with leather seats were provided for the studio, Eleanora placed a wooden drawing board over hers so she would remain disciplined.[8]

Eleanora's drawings presented both common conditions of the time—like ulcers, uterine prolapses, diverticulitis of the large intestine, tuberculosis of the spine, internal derangement of the knee, ectopic pregnancies, and horseshoe kidneys—and state-of-the-art procedures Mayo surgeons were pioneering, including hernia repair, radical mastectomies, tonsillectomies, splenectomies, and operations on the spinal cord. Her illustrations demonstrated precise control and a sense of draftsmanship for which Mayo artists ultimately became known. However, Eleanora's drawings were also distinctive. She expressed a "heightened sense of drama," pointing the viewer to a "single moment of great action, frozen in time, almost like the still scene editing of a suspense film."

In 1932, after twenty years as the head of the art studio at Mayo Clinic, Eleanora left. Her parents had died and the Depression was in full force. She first went to New Orleans and drew for Dr. Alton Ochsner at Tulane University before he started the Ochsner Medical Center. She worked there for three to four years before returning to New York City in her early fifties. Although

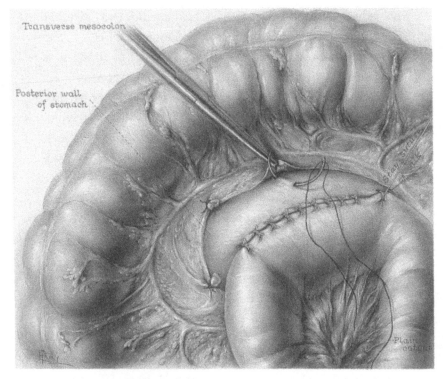

One of Eleanora Fry's drawings

little is known about her after that time, her drawings left a legacy of precision and artistry that had a lasting impact on medical illustration at Mayo and nationally. A critical study of her drawings was still a part of the standard medical illustration curriculum for half a century after she left Rochester.

In the same year that the clinic building opened, Dr. Gertrude Booker Granger changed roles. Dr. Charlie had been the Rochester public health officer since 1912, replacing a physician the public thought had been ineffective in combating scarlet fever. Dr. Booker Granger had been his assistant in the clinical practice, and in 1914 she became the deputy director of public health. Dr.

Charlie handled the political aspects of the job, and the Mayos provided office space and funding.

From 1914 to 1919, Dr. Booker Granger worked with Dr. Charlie to organize a system for collecting garbage, which was fed to hogs on a sixty-acre farm that Dr. Charlie purchased for productive recycling. Previously, garbage accumulated in city alleys and was collected on an irregular basis. They also worked on passage of an ordinance requiring inspection of milk, dairies, dairy herds, and bottling/pasteurizing plants. Pasteurization was considered an important step in preventing tuberculosis, a leading cause of death in the early 1900s, second only to pneumonia. The Civic League played a pivotal role in lobbying for these changes as well. Dr. Booker Granger's contributions to medicine now went beyond the significant work she had already done in ophthalmology.[9]

Dr. Booker Granger was not the only woman physician associated with the Mayos when the clinic building opened. By then Dr. Leda Stacy had been an integral part of the practice for six years.

After administering anesthesia at Saint Marys Hospital for two years, Dr. Stacy became a member of Dr. Christopher Graham's section of general internal medicine. In 1915, Dr. Will asked Dr. Stacy to study a new treatment, the use of radium, at Johns Hopkins University. Most of the medical work with radium, including intrauterine application for uterine myomas and menorrhagia, was being done on the East Coast. At the conclusion of her first trip, Dr. Stacy returned to Rochester with two tubes of radium. Over the next three years, she continued to travel to Philadelphia, Baltimore, and Boston to study the use of radium, especially applications in gynecology.[10]

Dr. Stacy became head of the section of radium therapy and led the intrauterine use of radium in the treatment of uterine myomas. As the use of radium expanded, a radium plant was opened in Rochester to assure a supply of radon seeds and tubes.

Dr. Leda Stacy

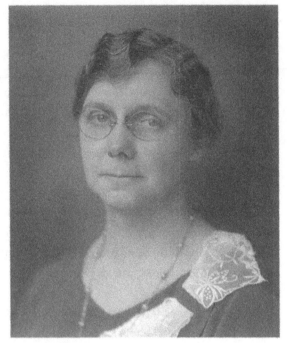

Dr. Stacy published many articles on radium therapy and became an internationally known and frequently quoted expert.

She continued in this role until 1917, when she was appointed head of a section with a special focus on gynecology, soon known as the Stacy section. The section was staffed with women associate staff members and men and women fellows. They consulted on gynecologic problems throughout the clinic and assured that any woman requesting a woman physician could be accommodated. As Dr. Stacy transferred out of Dr. Graham's area to begin her own section, Dr. Graham declared, "she is good, competent, and deserving... she goes from our department with regrets, but nonetheless with our willingness and joy for her." While her section was established to meet the needs of female patients, one woman complained, "I didn't come all the way from New York City to have a woman doctor warm her hands on me out here."

The Stacy section grew, adding four women physicians over the next few years.[11]

In 1913, Dr. Will Mayo received a letter from a physician in Galveston, Texas, introducing Dr. Georgine Luden, "a woman of remarkable attainments ... a very charming woman, very cosmopolitan, and of great intellectual force. She is a very wealthy woman in her own right, and has apparently taken up the study of medicine as a hobby. I feel certain you will find her extremely interesting and thoroughly emancipated. I hope you will be as favorably impressed with her as I have been."[12]

Dr. Luden was Dutch and educated first in Munich by some of the finest and most well-known physicians in Europe, including Friedrich v. Müller, Max v. Borst, and Emil Kraepelin. She was awarded the degree of MD summa cum laude at the University of Munich in 1911. As political tensions that eventually led to World War I intensified, she came to the United States, interested in conducting cancer research.[13]

In 1914, Dr. Luden arrived in Rochester on a train with an entourage of three staff—a cook, a maid, and a chauffeur/gardener—and two dogs named Toddy and Rowdy. She rented several rooms at the Zumbro Hotel but soon purchased a home.

During her voyage, a young woman from Kentucky had become ill. May Fisher was an aspiring opera singer who had recently enjoyed some success as the lead soprano in Wagner's *Tristan and Isolde* in the Berlin Opera House, a significant accomplishment for a young American singer. However, her health was declining and she, too, decided to leave Europe before war broke out. Hearing she was ill, Dr. Luden knocked on May's cabin door and asked if she could be of professional service. Out of this encounter, the two women became friends. Dr. Luden encouraged May to come to Rochester for medical care. Eventually, May visited Mayo Clinic for treatment of her gallbladder. At the same time, Dr. Luden was establishing her laboratory and needed staff. May became her laboratory assistant.[14]

During Dr. Luden's first year in Rochester, on July 15, 1915, Louise Wright Mayo died at eighty-nine years old. A few months earlier, she had slipped off a porch step one evening while calling her cat and broke her hip. Weeks of inactivity weakened her. She had attended the unveiling of a statue of her husband in June. Arriving in a wheelchair, she sat on stage with an umbrella held over her. She was living with Trude, her eldest daughter; Trude's son—Louise's grandson—David, now a physician with the Mayo practice, was the attending physician at her death.[15]

Her obituary, titled "Mrs. Louise Mayo Passes Away . . . After Life of Real Service," described her last moments, suggesting that death "came peacefully and calmly, the tired body relaxing, the spirit hovering for a moment and then taking its flight to realms eternal." The paper also noted that she lived her motto of being useful "until the day I drop." It continued, "When she had helped in giving of a commonwealth to civilization and been her husband's unwavering companion thru poverty and adversity, fire, famine and Indian warfare, to the days when she could enjoy all of life's comforts and live in the knowledge that she had given to the world men who were world famed as doers for mankind."[16]

Another local newspaper described her as "a woman of remarkable intellectual power, of wide reading, and charming personality." Louise left a legacy that grew to benefit scores of people across the globe. As remarkable as the Mayo practice was at the time of her death, fifty years after she and William came to Rochester for the first time, it was well on its way to being recognized as one of the finest and largest medical centers in the world.[17]

Dr. Luden's love of creative pursuits and May's singing talents inspired them to host teas and Sunday evening dinners. Their home became a salon for those interested in the arts and for many international visitors. While Dr. Luden was welcomed by many, some people became suspicious of her. Her Dutch accent was often mistaken for German, and some community members thought she and her staff might be spies and considered them "Enemy Aliens." Although Dr. Luden was fluent in English, Dutch, French, and German, she spoke to her Bavarian house staff in German, the only language they had in common. May sang patriotic songs at public meetings and was active in a civic committee organized to sell war bonds in an attempt to dispel animosity toward them.[18]

The following year, in 1916, Dr. Luden decided to have a carriage house built and contracted with a young recent graduate of Harvard University Graduate School of Design. Harold Crawford was a local man who had just returned to Rochester to open an architectural office. In the process of designing Dr. Luden's carriage house, he met May and they fell in love. In April 1917, a month after his twenty-ninth birthday, Harold Crawford entered military service. The United States was now involved in the war.[19]

While Harold was away, Dr. Luden encountered a woman from British Columbia who was terminally ill with breast cancer. The cancer was too advanced for her to survive, but she was pregnant, and Dr. Luden sought to keep the mother alive long enough to save the unborn child. She invited the woman to stay with her so she, May, and her staff could care for her. They were successful, and a baby girl was born on June 29, 1918. The mother, greatly weakened from the birth, named her daughter and handed the baby to May, telling her the baby was hers now. The woman's husband had no interest in the child, and the maternal grandmother later visited and agreed that the baby girl was best left with May. Harold Crawford was discharged from the army in January 1919. He and May married that September and subsequently adopted little Margaret.[20]

In addition to facing discrimination for her European ties and German-sounding accent, Dr. Luden struggled to retain her

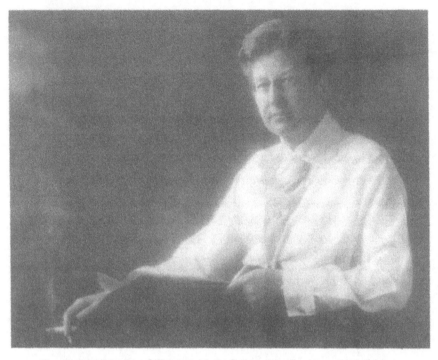

Dr. Georgine Luden, fully emancipated woman and cancer researcher

laboratory. The quickly growing clinic was running out of space downtown, and it was necessary to move her research out to Saint Marys Hospital. She was not pleased with the plan, worried that she would not have the same visibility and support located away from the clinic activities. Eventually, she relented and agreed to the move and continued her research. In addition to laboratory work, Dr. Luden incorporated epidemiological approaches into her research. For example, she marked a map of Rochester according to the coal pollution produced and numbers of cancer deaths in each neighborhood in order to investigate the potential correlation between the sulfur content of soft coal and cancer.[21]

Four years after the clinic building opened, in 1918, Hattie and Dr. Will moved out of their simple house and built a Tudor-style man-

sion on College Street. Hattie collaborated with the Ellerbe architectural firm, which had worked with Dr. Plummer on the clinic's
design. Hattie provided detailed drawings of the home she desired, which would balance the needs of her family with the capacity to entertain international guests, dignitaries, and large numbers
of visiting physicians. Dr. Will requested that a tower be included
for stargazing, in tribute to his mother's influence. The five-story
tower also included a simple, private study for Dr. Will to escape
to when the house was full of family and guests. The home, later
known as the Foundation House, was built on the highest hill in
Rochester and surrounded by elegant gardens. Hattie and Edith,
with her country home, were now both well established and prepared to manage the social aspects of their husbands' roles in the
growing and increasingly influential medical practice.[22]

The Mayo brothers were committed to education, which is no
surprise given their parents' attitudes about schooling. As early
as 1905, they initiated a three-year medical internship program

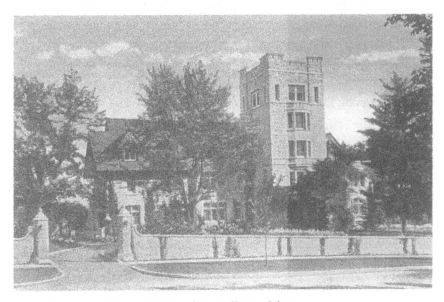

Foundation House, Hattie and Dr. Will Mayo's home

that focused mostly on laboratory and hospital rotations. Others came to study for shorter, six-month experiences. In 1915, the Mayos formalized an affiliation with the University of Minnesota. Many Mayo staff had received their degrees there, and Dr. Will had been a regent since 1907. The proposed arrangement included a $1.5 million gift to the university to support graduate medical education. The gift came from Drs. Will and Charlie, and from Hattie and Edith, since the accumulated fortune was theirs as well. This significant alliance with the university was intended to ensure that a sufficient number of students would have opportunities to obtain master's and doctoral degrees while completing clinical rotations at Mayo Clinic. The first class under the new arrangement consisted of four students, including two women, Della Gay Drips and Dorothy Foster Pettibone, who enrolled in 1915 and graduated in 1917. It was remarkable that this first class of graduate students was 50 percent women.[23]

Receiving her MS in pathology as a part of this first graduate class was the beginning of a long, successful career for Della Drips. She had already worked at Mayo as a laboratory assistant in the division of experimental surgery. Originally from La Crosse, Wisconsin, Della took courses in medicine at the University of Wisconsin in 1912, but during her studies she returned to Rochester, where her family then lived, to work in the Mayos' laboratories. Dr. Louis Wilson hired her in 1913, warning her not to think she was better than the other women working in the labs at the time, who had high school degrees. Dr. Wilson referred to his female lab staff as his "angels." The women in the lab quickly became friends, and Della found herself in a rich environment, where the women were permitted to listen to the staff physicians lecturing to young doctors. The women also taught each other.

Soon, Dr. Wilson asked Della to begin work at the experimental laboratory that was initially housed in his barn. She worked there with physicians and other staff until the laboratory was moved to the top floor of the clinic building, in part to be more

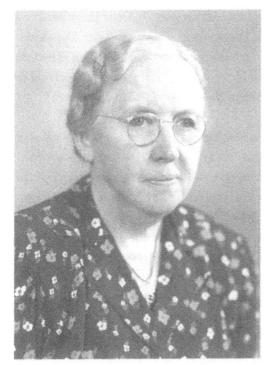

Dr. Della Drips

secure from anti-vivisectionists, the term at the time for animal rights activists. Their work involved studies of the thyroid gland, pancreas, and ovaries. They were also working diligently to develop sound practices for blood transfusion, needed not only for surgery but also on the war fronts in Europe. Della also studied ovulation in gophers with Dr. Frank Mann; their work resulted in findings important to understanding the cycles of the ovaries. At one point, Della traveled to learn laboratory slide fixing and staining techniques developed at the University of Chicago.

Having enrolled in the first class of graduate students at the University of Minnesota, Della was able to submit her work on ovulation as the thesis for her MS degree in 1917, which she followed by earning her MD in 1921. During her training, she was described as someone with "quiet power, accomplishing her routine duties, meeting emergencies and controlling the interns with no evident effort." In October of that year, Dr. Della Drips became a fellow at the clinic and began seeing women patients. She continued to have research interests and was considered an expert on gynecologic endocrinology. After a year, she was transferred to Dr. Stacy's section, where she was soon placed on the staff.[24]

In 1917, about the time Dr. Drips completed her master's degree, Hattie Mayo's new home was complete, Dr. Stacy was studying radium, and Dr. Luden was well into her cancer research at the clinic, the United States was involved in World War I. Base Hospital 26, a collaborative effort between the University of Minnesota and Mayo Clinic, also supported by the American Red Cross and private citizens, was organized. In 1918, the unit deployed to Allerey, France, with Mayo Clinic and University of Minnesota physicians, nurses, and a few laboratory technicians, secretaries, and other staff.

Drs. Will and Charlie were initially planning on deploying as well, but it was soon determined that it would be better to keep them safe at home in advisory roles. Eventually, they each attained the rank of brigadier general and spent considerable time in Washington, DC. Before war was declared, Dr. Will had been appointed chairman of the Committee of American Physicians for Medical Preparedness, which created a plan for fifty base hospitals that would be deployed if necessary. Each hospital would be fifty miles from the front lines and staffed with twenty-seven medical officers, sixty nurses, and 153 enlisted men. Base Hospital 26 was one of these units.[25]

The clinic remained busy during the war years, partially due to publicity from Drs. Will and Charlie's leadership in Washington and also because staff of all types were away from the clinic for military service, which meant the load doubled and tripled for those remaining at home. Dr. Charlie was also elected president of the American Medical Association during this period. The doctors' war, medical association, and clinic responsibilities became exhausting, and their health suffered. Dr. Will developed a severe case of jaundice, and Dr. Charlie came down with pneumonia. Their conditions frightened their families, as jaundice could have been a symptom of cancer, and pneumonia could be deadly in the pre-antibiotic era. Fortunately, both men recovered.[26]

Although the Mayo brothers were not deployed, many Mayo staff were, including twenty-nine-year-old Nora Guthrey, who had joined the editorial department in 1916. She had been born in Sioux Falls, South Dakota, and as a child moved with her family to Fort Collins, Colorado. She had a teaching certificate and experience teaching second grade. She married but was soon widowed. Her maternal grandparents lived in High Forest, a few miles south of Rochester. Presumably, she came to the area to be near them and found a position at the clinic.[27]

The clinic's administrator, Harry Harwick, described Nora as "dependable and efficient" in a letter of reference to the commander of Base Hospital 26. She was among personnel recruited for the unit in the summer of 1917, called to active duty in December, but not mobilized until the spring of 1918. In March, two hundred people were invited to a farewell reception for Nora and others. The event included an afternoon for ladies only, followed by an evening reception and program. Refreshments and music were provided throughout. The pastor of the Congregational church "made a few very appropriate remarks concerning the chaotic condition of countries and affairs and the need of loyal support, commending the efficient work of women when needed, from the time of Jeanne d' Arc to during the present crisis."[28]

Before the unit deployed, its members gathered at St. Paul's Episcopal Church, where their chaplain, Bishop W. P. Remington, addressed them.

[He] compared the position of the United States in the war to that of David going forth to meet the heavily

Nora Guthrey

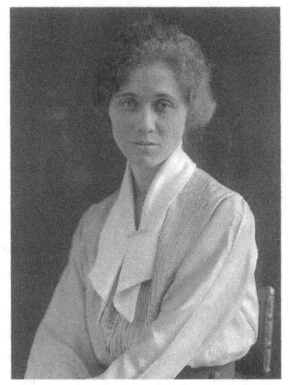

armed Goliath, but he spoke not of the war, but of the
need to deal with the devastation of war—to do everything that could be done to mitigate its horrors . . . it's
not a playday jaunt we are going on, for, though we are
not going to the firing line, we are enlisting for a service
which requires high courage, untiring energy and un-
bounded cheerfulness. Ministering to wounded men is
no easy task.[29]

In July 1918, when the unit reached Allerey, France, everyone,
including the thirty-six medical officers, fifty nurses, and two
hundred enlisted men with experience as carpenters, machinists,
plumbers, plasterers, undertakers, pharmacists, ambulance driv-
ers, tailors, barbers, stenographers, and clerks, pitched in to set

up the facilities. When they first arrived, very little was prepared. The ground was graded, but not much else had been done. When asked if they were ready to handle patients, their commander said, "I have beds, the food, the hands, and the best will in the world." Members of the unit improvised, "turning rough lumber, bricks, sheet iron, and roofing into bathing slabs, sterilizers, tables, chairs, and benches essential for the care of the wounded." On July 30, 1918, the first train of injured soldiers arrived and the staff evacuated the convoy in forty-three minutes, which French officials said was a record. Although Nora was assigned to clerical and laboratory technician duties, in this environment, she invariably filled in wherever she was needed.[30]

A dozen nurses from Rochester were among the hundred nurses in the unit, assisting in surgery and providing bedside care. The unit's two thousand beds were often full. Up to three trains of injured soldiers arrived at night. Two day nurses and one night nurse cared for wards with up to 118 patients. The beds were often twelve to sixteen inches apart. The nurses alternated the heads and feet of the beds to help deter the spread of infectious diseases. Influenza and diphtheria were of special concern, but meningitis, scarlet fever, measles, mumps, and respiratory illnesses, including pneumonia, were also evident. Inadequate heating and the damp, poorly ventilated wards may also have contributed to illness. War injuries included wounds from artillery, burns, and lung damage due to mustard gas exposure. The Rochester nurses were among 21,000 U.S. nurses who served at the peak of World War I, stationed in Hawaii, the Philippines, Puerto Rico, France, Italy, and Belgium. By the end of the war, one in three nurses in the country had served and over four hundred died from injuries and illnesses such as influenza and pneumonia.[31]

Upon their arrival in France, several of the Rochester nurses attached to Unit 26 were assigned to a mobile unit sent close to the front lines, where they prepared patients for transfer to hospital units. The Rochester-trained nurses were in high demand for the mobile units because of their surgical experience. One Rochester nurse, Nell Bryant, was assigned to Mobile Hospital 1, which received wounded servicemen directly from the trenches. Nell was originally from Monroe, Louisiana. As a nurse, she had escorted her aunt and uncle to Rochester in 1914 when her uncle required surgery. She returned to Rochester for three additional months of training and worked in anesthesia before joining the Red Cross, along with ten of her colleagues.[32]

Nell, writing to her sister, described hearing gunfire through the night but reported that she still felt protected and safe. She also affirmed her commitment to being there.

> I am just where I want to be, I wouldn't be back home for any thing on earth and knowing at the same time nurses are needed over here as badly as they are, every nurse in the U.S.A. should count it a great privilege to come over here and do her bit, we are specially trained and owe just as much to our Country and the boys are giving everything and we to [sic], should be willing to give our lives if need be.[33]

The unit's commanding officer issued a citation to his crew for "skill and a self-sacrificing devotion to duty that is beyond all praise." He gave special commendation to the nurses: "To the noble women nurses of this hospital, the Corps is especially indebted. They brought comfort and assistance to our wounded which none but women of such high attainments and ideals could administer. Their labors were an inspiration and they have written a new chapter in the annals of womanhood, which in future will be cherished by our people."[34]

After returning home, Nell was reunited with Dr. John Crenshaw, who was waiting for her. They had made the decision to deploy together, but he was assigned to a hospital in Newport News, Virginia, while she went overseas. He arrived back in Rochester first and made arrangements for them, including finding an apartment and furnishing it according to his taste, which, given that he was an avid hunter, included displaying moose heads in the living room. They were married on October 18, 1919.[35]

Other nurses with connections to Mayo Clinic also served in the war, including graduates of the Saint Marys School of Nursing, which had opened in 1906. One of these women, Florence Bullard from the class of 1913, became a Red Cross nurse assigned to Evacuation Hospital 13. She was the first American woman to be recognized by the French government for bravery. When the unit closed in January 1919, the head surgeon gave her the flag. She was awarded the Croix de Guerre and bronze star. The citation noted that her "devotion to her profession and bravery was greatly admired by all.... She showed the most imperturbable sang-froid under all the violent bombardments ... searching, in spite of the danger, for the wounded to assist and comfort them.... Her attitude was especially brilliant during the night of July 31, when bombs burst quite near the outpost." Solider poet Hardwicke Nevin wrote and dedicated the poem "Soissons" to Florence, "with tremendous admiration for her as a soldier and woman." The poem was published in the May 1920 issue of *Scribner's Magazine*.[36]

After the war, Florence returned to her hometown, Glen Falls, New York, and became the superintendent of nurses at Samuel and Nettie Bowne Hospital in Poughkeepsie. She stayed there through her retirement in 1954 but remained in close touch with the sisters at Saint Marys Hospital. In 1961, when her sight and health were declining, she sent the medal of bravery and citation to the sisters because her feeling was "they are not mine at all—but that surely they were presented to me in recognition of the Sisters of Saint Marys and their wonderful work in creating and carrying on the School of Nursing."[37]

Florence Bullard

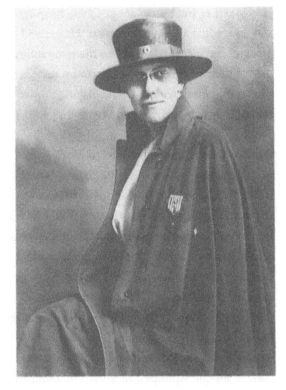

In addition to deployment, nurses were supporting the war effort at home by playing an instrumental role in anesthesia education. Mary Hines continued the quality practice begun by
Edith Graham Mayo and Alice Magaw. She had inherited their
reputations as one of the finest nurse anesthetists in the country.
The U.S. Army began sending groups of twenty nurses at a time
to study with her at Saint Marys Hospital, where six operating
rooms were used six days a week. Mary Hines and her colleagues
provided a six-week course, with each student administering anesthesia for fifty cases before she deployed to a unit overseas.[38]

Although the armistice was signed on November 11, 1918, Unit
26 remained in operation until January 10, 1919. More than 5,700
wounded and sick soldiers were cared for while it was open. After

her arrival home, Nora Guthrey received an invitation to a barbecue to "Welcome Our Boys." The card read, "You are one of 'Our Boys.' We are proud of you." On Nora's card, "Boys" was crossed out and "Girls" was written in.[39]

Nora resumed employment with Mayo Clinic, this time as Dr. Will's secretary. She remained in this role as his trusted partner until his death in 1939. For those twenty years, Nora competently handled his vast volume of correspondence and managed his calendar. Often she would need to reply on his behalf when he was away from the clinic. Few people would be prepared to expertly handle this responsibility for an internationally renowned medical leader.

After being Dr. Will's secretary, Nora remained employed at Mayo Clinic in various capacities. Most notably, she researched and wrote histories of early medical practitioners in the region, initially for the Minnesota Medical Society periodical *Minnesota Medicine*, and subsequently a collection of the histories was published in book form. She also served for two terms as president of the Olmsted County Historical Society and was involved in several community organizations.

While the war was being fought in Europe, influenza struck. Fifty million people died from the flu worldwide, far more than the sixteen million who died in the war. And Rochester was not immune. As the numbers of highly infectious patients grew, Sister Joseph and the Sisters of Saint Francis rose to the occasion. They purchased the nearby Lincoln Hotel and converted it into an isolation hospital in October 1917. The hospital filled almost immediately, with cots even being placed in hallways. In one day, eighteen nurses were admitted. With this shortage of trained staff, friends and relatives were called upon to help. Hattie Mayo's youngest daughter, Phoebe, was among them. By May 1918, when the menace had run its course, 360 patients had been hospitalized and forty-one had died.[40]

Despite these challenges, Mayo Clinic experienced the greatest period of growth in its history between 1912, when the serious planning of the new clinic building began, and the conclusion of World War I. The number of clinic patients doubled, to 60,000 annually, and 23,000 surgical procedures were performed. The union of forces that Dr. Will claimed as critical to serving the best interests of the patients in his 1910 graduation address at Rush Medical College was being actualized by many women filling a wide array of roles in the first decades of the practice. Their talents, expertise, and courage contributed to the clinic's success and to serving the best interest of patients at home and abroad.[41]

Further, woman suffrage became a reality during this period. On June 4, 1919, when many women were returning home from serving in the war, Congress passed the Nineteenth Amendment, affording women the right to vote. It took until August 26, 1920, for the amendment to be ratified by two-thirds of the states and become law. Susan B. Anthony's dream was fulfilled fourteen years after her death and forty-three years after she spoke in Rochester.

EXTENDING THE LONG ARM OF THE PHYSICIAN

1920–1926

In addition to directly providing medical care, women started new services to more holistically meet the needs of the patients and their families. They learned from what others were doing at other medical centers throughout the nation and quickly built upon the ideas, applying them to patient care delivery at Mayo Clinic and its related hospitals, which continued to grow.

As Mayo Clinic expanded in size and services, patients came to Rochester from greater distances and were increasingly diverse in nationality, ethnicity, and religion. Meeting their needs was more complex than serving an exclusively local population. Dr. Will, again with an eye to what other leading medical centers were doing, noted that the social needs of the patients were an important component to care and healing. Mayo Clinic's business manager, Harry J. Harwick, also felt that patients' financial concerns should be addressed.

Dr. Will and Hattie's daughter Phoebe and her friend Charlotte Bundy were students at Wellesley College, where Ida Cannon, chief of social services at Massachusetts General Hospital, inspired them to take a course in social work after graduation. Subsequently, Charlotte became ill and left the college, but in 1920, after graduation, Phoebe took a preliminary course in nursing at Saint Marys Hospital with another friend, Isabella Gooding. Dr. Will thought it advisable for anyone going into hospital work to "know the routine and how to protect themselves from contagious diseases." However, Phoebe soon met Dr. Waltman Walters, a young aspiring surgeon on the Mayo staff, and their marriage in 1921 preempted her career plans.[1]

Because both Dr. Will and Harry Harwick still felt there was a need for social work at the clinic, they contacted Phoebe's classmate Charlotte Bundy and offered to provide her with training in social work if she were still interested. Charlotte agreed and arrangements were made for her to spend time at Massachusetts General Hospital with Ida Cannon "to get the general idea of the thing." Years later, Charlotte wondered if Harry Harwick had any idea that within four years he would have not one but seven caseworkers, two secretaries, a librarian, and two occupational therapists on the payroll at the clinic.[2]

Charlotte visited Ida Cannon in Boston to learn more about social work, which was a growing, fairly well-established field on the East Coast. Ida had Minnesota connections. She grew up in St. Paul and completed nurse's training there in 1898, a year after Gertrude Booker graduated from University of Minnesota Medical School. Ida then worked as a nurse at the State School for the Feeble-minded in Faribault, Minnesota, Maud Mellish's hometown for two years.

Ida's nursing experience motivated her to expand her education in sociology and psychology. While taking courses at the University of Minnesota, she heard a talk given by Jane Addams, founder of the Hull House, a settlement house for immigrants in Chicago. Years later, Addams would be the first American woman awarded the Nobel Peace Prize, and she would be considered the founder of social work. Hearing Jane Addams speak motivated Ida to begin coursework in social work in Boston, and she eventually established the first social work department at Massachusetts General Hospital. Charlotte Bundy was learning about the field from the nation's leading expert.[3]

Before a formal social work service was organized, Willa Murray and Cora Olson staffed a desk in the lobby of the clinic building, primarily intended to assist the many young women working there with social needs such as housing and entertainment. Soon patients began coming to this desk seeking assistance in finding lodging or employment. During World War I, the staff also did some Red Cross work.[4]

In 1921, when Charlotte Bundy returned from Boston, she and another classmate, Isabella Gooding, who had also taken the preliminary nursing course at Saint Marys, set up a desk in the Colonial Hospital, which had opened in 1915 to help meet the increasing patient demand. The women began by conducting a survey of the patients and their needs while "performing friendly services for this group, such as writing letters, doing errands, providing reading material." From the survey, they learned that 51 percent of the patients arrived at Mayo Clinic without a family member to support them during their care. They subsequently began two primary initiatives: first, group work, largely recreational, to raise the patient's morale, and, second, casework, endeavoring to aid the physician in providing the best medical service possible.[5]

From the survey, Charlotte also recorded some of her most memorable contacts with patients she visited during the first months of her career. A Danish woman from Iowa was at the clinic alone. Her husband farmed and was unable to accompany her. She had come for an operation to treat goiter, a relatively common condition in the Midwest until iodized salt was discovered to resolve most cases. Charlotte found the woman in her room "throwing herself about the bed like a restless cricket." The patient was terribly worried and homesick. She stated she would rather go home that day and die rather than stay and wait for her treatment. Charlotte found Danish books for the woman to read and arranged for a Danish couple in town to visit her regularly. At the conclusion of her three-week stay, the surgeon noted in her medical record that they would not have been able to keep the patient in town for her operation if it had not been for the "efforts of the social worker."[6]

Children arriving alone for care were of particular concern. One girl about twelve years old was sent on the train from Montana with a note pinned on her frock that read, "Please be good to this little girl. She is going to the Mayo Clinic." Charlotte noted that one "very public spirited County nurse from North Dakota . . . was rounding up children" with congenital dislocated hips, including a pair of four-year-old twins who were county charges, and bringing them to Rochester for care. Charlotte found boarding places for the children to stay while they recuperated in their plaster casts. She soon acquired a Model T car for transporting patients and "loads of books from the library." One nine-year-old girl from a large, poor farm family loved the individual attention and rode around in the Model T with Charlotte, sharing her happy nature and joy with those they visited.

Sometimes a whole family came to Rochester, which created different demands. Charlotte documented the case of a family from the McKenzie River Valley of the Canadian Northwest who traveled thousands of miles first by dogsled, then ship, and finally train. One of the children reported that due to the remoteness of their home, they had never seen children other than Eskimos or worn shoes other than moccasins before.

Due to the "tremendous demand" for books, Isabella Gooding started a community drive. Initially, the Rochester Public Library provided books, but the numbers were becoming unsustainable. The newspaper reported the appeal with the headline, "Here's Your Chance to Help a Worthy Cause, So Get Busy." During "Hospital Book Week," Rochester residents were encouraged to donate books to support healing. The social workers provided a list of books that were in demand, including titles by Edna Ferber, Zane Grey, Sinclair Lewis, and Jack London. Another newspaper article commented on the medicinal impact books can have: "war has shown us the value of intelligent use of books in connection with hospital work. Many an ex-service man can point to very real and practical benefit, educational as well as therapeutic which the camp library rendered him."[7]

Over a thousand books were collected from the public drive, and physicians and their families donated as well. A couple of librarians employed by Rochester Public Library but whose salaries were paid by the clinic obtained special training in Minneapolis. The arrangement continued until 1946, when the hospital library service became part of the clinic library and Ruth Tews, chief of the hospital library department at the St. Paul Public Library and director of the hospital librarianship course at University of Minnesota, was hired. She expanded the services and promoted bibliotherapy, reading as a means for healing. The librarians chose books that would entertain and, more importantly, divert the patient's attention outward, away from discomfort and problems.[8]

Physicians began to clamor for social workers to see their patients—all of their patients, not just a few of them. They quickly realized the benefit of having this unit care for the patient's social, psychological, and financial concerns so that physicians could focus on the patient's medical needs. Social workers were considered the "long arm" of the physician in this regard. A team approach could greatly expedite and enhance care and recovery. In their first months, Charlotte Bundy and another social worker made between three hundred and five hundred patient visits a month in the Colonial Hospital alone.[9]

Certain health conditions required more attention because of the length of treatment, the need for post-hospitalization planning, and other social issues. Pulmonary tuberculosis and syphilis "were rampant and the streets were filled with patients with post operative goiter dressings."[10]

For tuberculosis patients, social workers at Mayo Clinic followed an extensive eight-step protocol developed to address the infectious, debilitating, and financially draining nature of the disease. They were responsible for reporting the patient's diagnosis to the local health officials and boardinghouse, so the room could be thoroughly cleansed after the patient left. They interviewed the patient to form an impression of his or her "understanding of and attitude toward" the diagnosis, reviewed the patient's social situation, gave instruction on proper hygiene, and helped make arrangements for treatment at sanatoriums. They followed up with the patient and the patient's home physicians for two to three months. The tuberculosis diagnosis brought with it a great financial burden as well. Case reports show situations where a newly diagnosed young farmer was distraught because he was married, had three children to support, and had recently bought a farm. Social workers were in contact with sanatoriums, health boards, and relief agencies throughout the country in their efforts to assist these patients. Their files included contact information for several hundred public health nurses nationwide.[11]

Cases of syphilis were equally challenging. One young woman from Alberta, Canada, came to Rochester for treatment for inherited syphilis that had affected her sight. Doctors at Mayo thought her situation could be improved and her vision saved, but it would take three to five years. Due to her poor sight, her education had been limited, and she could not read or write. The social worker found her work as a chambermaid at the hospital and a room in a boardinghouse, where she could also work for her room and board. The social worker also arranged for her to take Americanization classes at the high school to resume her education. After a year, the patient had earned enough money to pay her own medical costs and send her sister, who was also not well, a train ticket to join her in Rochester.

Financial support for patients with venereal diseases was challenging because many churches and community organizations were not receptive to helping. Some young, unmarried women who had contracted syphilis or were pregnant were helped to enroll in courses for vocations like hairdressing and stenography, so they could eventually support themselves and pay for their treatment. On at least one occasion, the social worker sought past-due alimony from a patient's first husband to help cover the costs of her and her daughter's care after conducting an investigation that revealed he was the likely origin of the patient's condition.[12]

Assisting syphilis patients required social workers to be nonjudgmental and to focus on the patients' well-being. They were integrally involved in educating patients and families on the condition and its cause. And they were often the ones to have conversations with patients about providing the names of past sexual partners, which was not an easy subject to broach, especially at that time. Some patients were so ill that treatment was not feasible, and the whole family had to adjust to the hardships of their disabled state. The nerves in one man's legs were damaged to the point he could not work, but the social workers arranged for him to learn to hook rugs as a way to pass time. In the worst situations, the syphilis was advanced to the point of causing insanity, and social workers committed patients to a state hospital. The social workers also helped patients with any venereal disease to deal with the isolation caused by their diagnosis, knowing they could not as easily talk with others about it, as well as deal with the consequences, financial implications, and emotional impact of this socially unacceptable diagnosis.[13]

Unmarried mothers faced similar social stigma and financial anxieties. The social work section developed a policy to assure that the "interests and opportunities of these girls may be recognized and developed and the interests of the children born illegitimately may be safe-guarded."[14]

In 1923, Juliet Eisendrath was hired to assist Jewish patients to "bridge the gap" between themselves and the clinic. At that time there were between fifty and seventy-five Jewish patients hospitalized and fourteen hundred patients were coming to the clinic annually for treatment, many of them orthodox in their beliefs. Those who spoke Yiddish often felt "bewildered and lost" in the "rush and routine of a large organization."

Juliet claimed that the Jewish patient is "high strung and sensitive and very often misunderstands the acts and words of the staff," and noted that treatment under these circumstances is often "ineffective and progress impeded." Juliet noted that "many of the perplexities that otherwise loom up so formidably... could be explained by someone of their own kind." In addition to interpreting, Juliet assisted Jewish patients in finding appropriate housing and kosher meals. After her appointment, cross-cultural communication was improved and the clinic discontinued its practice of charging Jews, blacks, and Greeks a hundred-dollar deposit before rendering care. Juliet helped physicians understand Jewish diets and amend dietary recommendations to fit within their restrictions. She also advocated for the local Jewish community, then about twenty-five families, to assist in overall care of the Jewish patients, including visiting them in the hospital and proper disposition of the deceased.[15]

To facilitate healing and alleviate stress among patients due to finances, the occupational therapy program evolved quickly within the social work section. Priscilla Keely, Isabella Gooding, and Charline Buck sought to provide creative activities for ambulatory patients that would "occupy their time" and provide "something to do with their hands." Instruction in basketry, beading, and knitting was provided. The program quickly grew, and Beatrice Hardy, a graduate of the Boston School of Occupational Therapy, was hired to lead it. In addition to procuring supplies and providing instruction to patients, she trained nurses so they could assist patients at bedside. Some of the articles patients made were put up for sale, helping defray the costs of their care. The occupational therapists hoped patients, hospital staff, and the public would see the tangible outcomes of hours "usefully spent, in contrast to those spent in inactivity which always results in forming habits of idleness and self pity."[16]

In the early 1920s, many ex-servicemen were patients. One man spent several months in the hospital and then needed to remain in the area, but only for dressing changes and to have his condition monitored. After he was discharged from the hospital, he tried to find work but had too little endurance for the available jobs. The social services section directed him to the occupational therapy shop, where he was taught to make rakes for scarf making. The rakes were sold in the gift shop and the proceeds helped support the patient. He then began making toys out of wood, which were also sold on his behalf. He eventually left Rochester happy to have learned a trade he could use at home in California.[17]

The occupational therapy program quickly outgrew the spaces allocated to it in the various hospitals. In 1925 the "Little Green House" was purchased downtown near the Colonial and Worrell Hospitals and the clinic building. For thirty-one years, this brick house painted a dull green with pale yellow and pumpkin-red blinds housed the occupational therapy program. It was a charming place with a fireplace and homey living room and a garden in the back yard with a large oak tree. Staff felt it provided patients with "an oasis in a desert of hospitals, laboratories and boarding houses."

The director of this new initiative, Beatrice Hardy, soon met and, in 1926, married Dr. Arthur Desjardins. When Harry Harwick was interviewing candidates for her replacement, he asked repeatedly, "Are you interested? Are you interested?" One of the women hired recalled her interview and realized throughout her career that "only by having a group of interested persons, interested in the ideals of the Mayo Clinic, interested enough to give of themselves . . . could the Clinic function so smoothly and successfully."[18]

The Little Green House provided space for recreational activities as well as occupational skill development. Halloween and Christmas parties were held there; motion pictures were shown.

The staff even provided a marionette presentation of "Jack and the Bean Stalk," which became quite popular. A supervisor felt compelled to assure the other staff that the therapists had written the script and built the dolls and stage entirely on their own time and not during working hours.

Shortly after its inception, the occupational therapy department became independent of the social work section to better meet its unique mission. It quickly grew in size and reputation. A film documenting the activities at the Little Green House, including commentary by physicians and clips of recovering patients, was shown nationally and internationally to demonstrate the therapeutic techniques being used.

The first "Hospital Social Service Bulletin" of 1923 gave a glimpse into the working lives of the social workers by proposing that they each adopt two New Year's resolutions:

> *First* That each of us keep strictly to our hours. For the sake of principal [*sic*] we should not be caught within hospital walls in the evenings or our Saturday afternoons off, except in emergencies. We cannot be fair to either our work or ourselves if we continue with the prevailing custom of an unlimited working day . . .

> *Second* That all records of the past year be brought up to date by the first of February. It is believed that the painful performance of such a task will naturally result in a third resolution, to keep the new year records up to date as we go along.[19]

Not only did Charlotte Bundy and the social workers provide excellent patient care; they supported graduate education in their field. In 1926, the University of Minnesota director of the social work program proposed six-month fieldwork rotations at Mayo under the supervision of one of the clinic's social workers, Helen Anderson Young, who had trained in Boston and worked at medical centers in Chicago and Minneapolis before coming to Rochester. She had been lecturing regularly for two years at the University of Minnesota and was considered highly qualified. The subsequent rotations became one of several early allied health professional and nursing programs at Mayo Clinic committed to assuring a supply of well-educated staff into the future.[20]

The beginnings of the social work section were not without challenges. At least one social worker who was formally trained and experienced in social work resented Charlotte Bundy's supervisory role. Concerns about low salaries were expressed, causing one staff member to request salary survey information from the national professional association. Initial funding for the section came from Harry Harwick's administrative budget, some of which was derived from the proceeds of the Coca-Cola and milk machines throughout the clinic. Subsequently, it became a regularly budgeted function, and generous patients with financial resources donated funds for other patients who could not afford their care, medication, or living expenses during treatment.[21]

Working so closely together, many of the women in the section became like a family. Several rented apartments together, although it was unusual for "young ladies to live unchaperoned. They were careful to do nothing that could be criticized. They did not even sew on Sunday." Charlotte Bundy felt it would not be possible to "imagine a happier, richer experience for a group of young women wanting to serve their communities" and that the "family atmosphere of warmth and generous encouragement came down ... from the very top." Dr. Will Mayo complimented their work, and he and Hattie entertained them in their home.[22]

In 1927, Charlotte Bundy's leadership of the social work section ended when she married Dr. James Learmonth, a fellow training

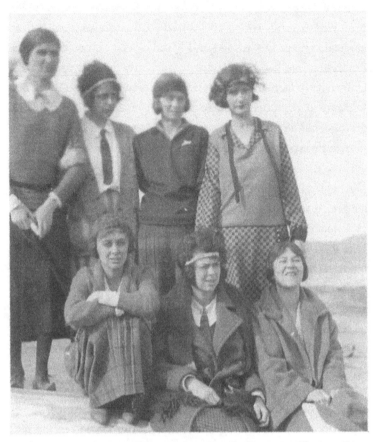

Front row, seated left to right: Charlotte Bundy (Learmonth), Priscilla Keely, Beatrice Hardy (Desjardins). Second row, left to right: Isabel Farr, Charline Buck, Ruth Rockwell (Schultz), Juliet Eisendrath (Cohen)

at the clinic. She moved with her husband to his homeland, Scotland, where he became well known and was appointed surgeon to the king and queen, resulting in knighthood. Priscilla Keely, who had joined the section as a social worker in its first year, became the director, a position she would hold for twenty-six years. During Charlotte's brief tenure, she started the section without formal training and developed it into a staff of seven social workers and six secretaries and desk attendants, in addition to the librarians and occupational therapists. She and her colleagues, all of them women—except for one man who provided workshop activities for men—established world-class social services for Mayo Clinic patients.[23]

Shortly after Priscilla Keely became director, another service was added to the section. Interpreters were often needed for foreign patients as well as for immigrants who were not fluent in English. There was a regular call for Polish and Italian interpreters and occasional calls for French, Greek, and Finnish assistance, in addition to the Yiddish translations already provided by the Jewish social worker. Because of the high volume of Spanish patients, an entire section at the clinic was devoted to their needs.[24]

The international practice had grown rapidly as Mayo Clinic's reputation extended beyond U.S. borders, driven by extensive publication of research and clinical findings under Maud Mellish Wilson's leadership and through affiliations with international medical societies and institutions. Drs. Will and Charlie and other Mayo physicians traveled extensively.

But Mayo Clinic's reputation specifically among Spanish-speaking countries soared in 1922 when Dr. Will saved the life of a well-known matador while the guest of the president of Mexico. During a bullfight they attended, the matador was badly gored, and the president asked Dr. Will if there was anything he could do. Dr. Will examined the bleeding man and was able to stop the hemorrhaging after the local doctors had been unsuccessful. The news of Dr. Will's impressive deed spread throughout Mexico and a good portion of Latin America. This incident, along with the good relations he had established when as president of the American College of Surgeons he had encouraged interactions with Latin American surgeons, including touring through several major South American countries in 1920, resulted in large numbers of Spanish-speaking patients from all walks of life coming to Rochester for treatment. A patient from Peru began donating books written in Spanish so these patients would have

Beatriz Montes

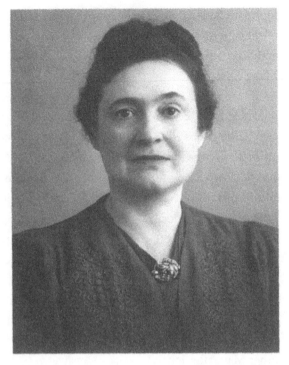

something to do while they were in town. Other donations came in, and soon an extensive Spanish library with a thousand volumes existed.[25]

Beatriz Montes came to Mayo Clinic as a patient in 1924, traveling from her home in Havana, Cuba. She was a graduate of Northfield Seminary in Massachusetts and had taught Spanish literature and history in Havana. During her recovery in Rochester, she assisted other Spanish-speaking patients by translating for them and making them feel welcome.

Because of her kind and generous nature, Beatriz Montes was hired by Mayo Clinic in 1925 to be an interpreter and the librarian for the Spanish collection. After twenty-six years of service in this role, she died in a fall during a power outage in her apartment building in 1951. In a display of appreciation, her colleagues dedicated a bilingual illuminated memorial scroll in the Spanish library with these words: "In memory of Beatriz Montes . . . who for twenty-six years by her insights into the minds and hearts of Latin Americans and North Americans facilitated their mutual regard, her friends have caused these words to be inscribed in the two languages which she spoke with equal grace."[26]

During the 1920s and '30s, many patient needs beyond the strictly medical were identified and met. Most of these services, also considered critical to a patient's successful recovery, were provided by women. Social workers, librarians, occupational therapists, and interpreters became recognized as important members of the care team.

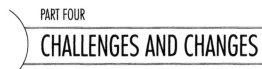

PART FOUR

CHALLENGES AND CHANGES

MEETING THE EXPANDING NEEDS

1922–1927

The steady increase in patients required expanded facilities, especially in the number of hospital beds and surgical suites. The Sisters of Saint Francis, with Sister Joseph at the helm, repeatedly rose to the occasion. Additional formally educated nurses were also required to staff the expansions, and nursing schools were opened to meet the need. Another new field, dietary services, was added during this period. All of these efforts were led by competent, intrepid, innovative women.

———

Sister Joseph had already spearheaded expansions at Saint Marys Hospital financed by the Sisters of Saint Francis in 1894, 1898, 1904, 1909, and 1912. This growth added operating rooms, laboratory space, and a maternity ward and brought the total number of beds to three hundred from the original twenty-seven. Yet it was not enough. By the hospital's twenty-fifth anniversary in 1914, over eight thousand individuals were being treated annually as inpatients, a substantial increase from three hundred patients a year earlier on. The need to care for more patients grew almost every year.[1]

In 1915, with a large facility to manage, Sister Joseph stepped down from her role as Dr. Will's surgical assistant. She had assumed this responsibility early in her career at Saint Marys in addition to being hospital superintendent. Dr. Will chose her over physicians to assist him because of her skillfulness in surgery. For twenty-five years, she stood at Dr. Will's side in the operating room, often in front of a galley full of visitors. Dr. Will trusted her

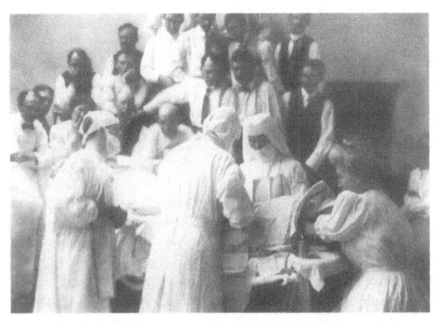

Right to left: Alice Magaw in surgery with Sister Joseph Dempsey and Dr. Will Mayo

to continue the procedures while he paused to address the audience: "Her fingers flew like magic and often, before they knew it, the operation was over." During her time as his assistant, with her fine sense of touch, she identified an umbilical nodule that was often the only sign of abdominal cancer. It was named "Sister Joseph's nodule," a nomenclature that has endured in surgical journals for nearly a hundred years.[2]

The need for additional hospital beds for the clinic practice seemed insatiable. In addition to Saint Marys, other privately owned hospitals opened in Rochester between 1907 and 1921: the Kahler, Colonial, Stanley, Worrell, Curie, and Damon Hospitals. By 1921, one thousand hospital beds and nineteen operating rooms in Rochester were dedicated to serving Mayo Clinic patients.[3]

And there was still need for more hospital beds and operating rooms. Sister Joseph and the Sisters of Saint Francis came for-

ward with a seven-story expansion completed in 1922, which provided three hundred additional beds and ten additional operating
rooms at a cost of $2.2 million, bringing the total capacity of Saint
Marys Hospital to nearly six hundred beds, making it the largest
privately owned hospital in the United States. An amphitheater
that could seat an audience of two hundred students and visiting
physicians was added into one of the operating rooms.[4]

The opening of the new surgical building took place on Hospital
Day, May 12, 1922, an annual celebration of Florence Nightingale's
birth. The Bureau of Retail Dealers in Rochester unanimously
agreed that all places of business would close from 4 to 6 PM so
that everyone could have an opportunity to attend the opening
celebrations. Festivities began that sunny spring day at 11 AM,
when the Rochester Civic and Commerce Association and other
dignitaries came to congratulate the sisters while Knutzen's Orchestra played in the sun parlor. Within the first two hours, over a
thousand people toured the new facility, and Rochester police officers were necessary to direct traffic. Admission tickets were sold

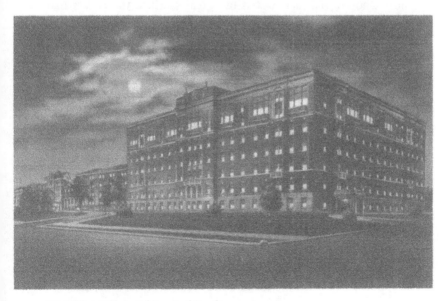

Saint Marys Hospital Surgical Pavilion, 1922

for twenty-five cents, with the proceeds benefitting the child welfare association. In total, four thousand people toured the facility and $990 was raised for the good cause.[5]

At 6:30 PM, dinner was served to distinguished guests, including the bishop, the mayor of Rochester, and other civic representatives and prominent Mayo physicians who offered congratulatory remarks. Dr. Henry Plummer noted, "only some one of great genius and great faith would dare to double the size of this already great hospital. The Sisters of Saint Francis did it. The genius, faith, and vision of Sister Joseph put this big thing through. She had the vision and greatness to do it."

Dr. Louis Wilson noted that other hospitals are not as successful because they lack what "the Sisters' lives have stood for,— womanly kindness." He also wondered how they would find enough "other women with the same spirit of kindness, women who will devote themselves, their lives, and their personal interests to the personal welfare of the individual patient."

A local pastor, the Reverend W. W. Bunge of the Evangelical Church of Peace, noted the great sacrifice the sisters had made: "Look at the farmer . . . he puts one kernel of corn into the ground; that one kernel sacrifices its existence and out of this sacrifice there comes forth a stalk . . . that bears fruit. Pluck the ear of corn and count the kernels. You will find that the average ear has seven hundred kernels that owe their life to that one kernel that sacrificed itself for them. Friends, I know that the existence and growth of Saint Marys Hospital are due to sacrifice, to great sacrifices made by the Sisters of Saint Francis."[6]

Dr. Will Mayo gave the greatest compliment of all:

We of the staff have been guided by her [Sister Joseph], and this institution, and her faith. . . . After all, the building is not the only necessary thing. A building is composed of brick and mortar, so to speak; but it is the ideals and the spirit that the building shelters, the ideals and spirit within it, that make the building great. What we accomplish in the future will not be due to the brick and mortar but to the soul and spirit that reside within Saint Mary's Hospital.

The dignitaries that evening also wanted Sister Joseph to speak during the banquet, but she sat off to the side, refusing to rise until the audience's applause drew her to the podium. Her comments were brief: "My very dear Friends: I do not deserve plaudits given to me tonight, but I will take them to distribute them among the Sisters with whom I have worked so many years to make Saint Mary's Hospital a house of God and a gateway to heaven for His many suffering children."

After the speeches and the last of the tours, "about half past ten the guests departed and as the long line of cars quietly left from the hospital grounds, a full-orbited moon was rising over Saint Mary's Hill to make glorious the night of a perfect day."

Sister Joseph had been administrator of the hospital for thirty-three years, and she was sixty-six years old at the time of the opening of the surgical building, but her tenure was far from over. She would serve for another seventeen years.

During her administration, Sister Joseph articulated some of her values in "Hospital Economy." In this article, she explained where hospitals should look for opportunities to economize and places where they should restrain from cutting budgets. Her guiding principal was, "We should provide for our patients better than the best home could do. In justice we owe them intelligent, scientific, efficient service; we must be willing to make sacrifices for their welfare. Our patients must be our first consideration and what is conducive to their health, comfort and convenience must be provided at any cost. Hospitals should not be boarding houses." In the article, she covers everything from utility and food expenses to finding qualified help and managing miscellaneous supplies. She knew the hospital business from top to bottom and was probably the most experienced hospital administrator in the country.[7]

The need for more hospital beds meant the need for more nurses. Sister Joseph realized this as early as 1906. The Sisters of Saint Francis also served as teachers, and she knew they did not have the capacity to continue providing enough sisters to meet the growing call for nurses. Further, the sisters who desired to be nurses needed formal training because nursing was evolving as a profession.

In 1906, Anna Jamme, a graduate of the Johns Hopkins School of Nursing, came to Saint Marys Hospital as a visitor to learn more about how nursing was being practiced at Mayo Clinic. Sister Joseph noticed that Anna remained intently focused during the two-hour operation she observed, taking notes the entire time. Sister Joseph took her on a tour of the hospital afterward and detected her passion and competence. Further, Anna was a devout Catholic. Some of the patients and Mayo Clinic doctors felt that the religious commitment and devotion of the sisters could not be replicated by lay nurses. Sister Joseph decided Anna Jamme was the one to start a school of nursing at Saint Marys Hospital.[8]

Anna Jamme agreed and became the first superintendent of the Saint Marys Hospital Training School for Nurses, later known as the Saint Marys School of Nursing. Two students were admitted in 1906, four in 1907, and ten in 1908. The two-year program was established with no tuition, and students received room and board at no charge, first in a cottage nearby and later in the motherhouse. The intention was to provide rooms for them at the hospital, but every bed was usually needed for patients. In exchange for tuition and room and board, they worked long hours in the hospital units and operating rooms. They took 142 hours of coursework in anatomy, bacteriology, physiology, and surgical

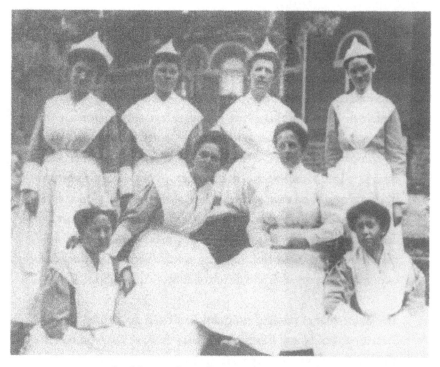

Anna Jamme, third from right, and 1906–07 nursing students

diseases. Most of the classes were provided in the evening, and nurses-in-training were required to study on the weekends.[9]

Although Anna Jamme left Rochester in 1911 to care for her mother in Poughkeepsie, New York, she gave the school an excellent start. Her devotion to the students and patients was often noted. She was a competent and compassionate mentor for the aspiring nurses. She also had the organizational skills and vision that Sister Joseph sought in an educational leader. Even after leaving Saint Marys, Anna Jamme continued her work, publishing articles on nursing education and an important textbook. She also contributed to the establishment of the Army School of Nursing in 1918.[10]

In an address to the alumni of the school in 1919, Dr. Will

Mayo acknowledged that at first he and others were skeptical about training lay women to be nurses rather than staffing the hospital entirely with sisters. They were concerned that lay nurses would be less efficient, but they were convinced otherwise. He announced that the nursing profession was just beginning its "great usefulness" and said that group medicine is necessary because "it is impossible for any man to know more than a little of what is to be known that will benefit the sick. . . . It therefore becomes necessary [to] act in unison, and in these groups of people devoted to the prevention and cure of disease, the nurse is destined to hold a very high place. . . . Much of the work done by the doctor can be done as well or better by the nurses." He further predicted a "brilliant future" for them and that they would "carry the principles of humanity, sympathy, and devotion to duty throughout life."[11]

The Saint Marys nursing program had been accredited by the State Board of Nurse Examiners in 1915. In 1916, 149 women applied to the program. Fifty were accepted and thirty-three eventually graduated, demonstrating the rigor of the program and the dedication required to complete it. The need for applicants to be responsible extended to their appearance. Women with bobbed hair were not admitted in the 1920s for fear that they would look too frivolous. In 1934, the admissions requirements noted that all students needed to be of certified good character. They also needed certification of their health by a physician. Students were to be within ten pounds of normal weight, not over or under weight, even though being underweight was considered fashionable at the time. Applicants needed to be between nineteen and thirty-five years old and unmarried. Some widows were admitted, but never divorcées. Students were also required to take swimming classes and obtain Red Cross life-saving certification to be ready for any emergency. With eighty students admitted annually in this three-year program, over two hundred students were on campus taking classes and caring for patients. By 1934, students had come from thirty-nine states and Cuba, China, the Philippines, and Panama.[12]

Eventually the facilities for the nursing school also grew. A dormitory was built in 1912 with capacity to house a hundred nurses. In 1927, another wing was added, bringing the capacity to three hundred students. The new facility was intended to be as homelike as possible, with rooms decorated in cream and light brown. A swimming pool, recreation hall, tea room, and laundry facility were included. In addition, a two-story auditorium was built with a seating capacity of twelve hundred and an elaborate pipe organ. The first use of the facility was in October 1927, when Dr. Charlie Mayo addressed 650 delegates of the American Hospital Association. During the program, the Saint Marys Nursing Student Orchestra and a professor of organ music at the University of Minnesota played selections from Donizetti, Sibelius's *Finlandia*, and other popular classical pieces. Although primarily for educational needs, the auditorium was the largest in Rochester at the time, and the sisters also made it available for civic gatherings, including Rochester Symphony performances.[13]

The sisters with years of nursing experience were the school's faculty, and those interested in becoming nurses also began enrolling in the program rather than being assigned to the hospital and trained on the job. Sister Domitilla, born Lillian DuRocher in Monroe, Michigan, was among the sisters to enroll, beginning the program in 1915 and graduating in 1918. An excellent student, she pursued a bachelor's degree and teaching diploma at Teachers College at Columbia University in New York. She became an educational director and science instructor in the Saint Marys nursing program in 1920. In 1934, she returned to Columbia for a master's degree, which she completed in 1935. She also contributed to the establishment of a graduate program in nursing at St. Teresa College, organized by the Sisters of Saint Francis in nearby Winona, Minnesota.[14]

Sister Domitilla
DuRocher

Students appreciated Sister Domitilla's teaching ability. They claimed, "If you could not learn Anatomy and Physiology from Sister Domitilla, you could not learn Anatomy and Physiology." Sister Domitilla enjoyed teaching that course the most, but often she was called upon to teach chemistry and ethics. And there was more in store for Sister Domitilla. In 1937, she was appointed assistant superintendent of Saint Marys Hospital and began administrative duties under the guidance of Sister Joseph, then eighty-one years old.[15]

The Saint Marys School of Nursing was not the only program in Rochester. Kahler Corporation, which owned five hospitals and was planning a sixth in 1920, also got into the business of training nurses and opened the Colonial School of Nursing, later renamed the Kahler Hospitals School of Nursing. Irene English, president of the State Registered Nursing Board, became director of the school in 1923. These two nursing schools affiliated with Mayo Clinic taught common methods. In 1920, the Saint Marys School of Nursing published a textbook, *The Operating Room: Instructions for Nurses and Assistants*, which both schools adopted. The unique methods meant that one could walk into an operating room anywhere in the country and tell if it was under the charge of a nurse who had graduated from a school affiliated with Mayo Clinic.[16]

Nearly all of the graduates of Saint Marys School of Nursing were hired at facilities other than Saint Marys Hospital. Under the supervision of the sisters, students provided a significant amount of patient care during their training, keeping personnel costs low, a practice typical in hospitals during this period but eventually concerning for nursing educators. Since the Kahler Corporation was staffed by lay people, not sisters of a religious order, some of its graduates were hired there, but both schools' mission was to provide a high-caliber nursing program for women and meet the staffing needs of hospitals throughout the nation.

Rochester was a mecca for nursing education. In addition to the Saint Marys and Kahler programs, the city was home to a third school of nursing. The Second State Hospital for the Insane, which had opened in Rochester in 1879—ten years before Saint Marys Hospital was launched—started a nursing program in 1889 and graduated sixteen nurses in 1892, including four men. Men were not admitted to the Saint Marys School of Nursing until 1937.[17]

Not only were more hospital beds and nurses needed; there was a need to expand patient services. About the same time Charlotte Bundy and her colleagues were organizing social services and occupational therapy, dietary programs were being developed. In October 1920, Mary Foley came to Rochester to assume leadership of the dietetics program for Mayo Clinic patients. Originally from Worchester, Massachusetts, she attended Pratt Institute in

Brooklyn from 1911 to 1913 and subsequently held dietary positions in Cleveland, Ohio, and Augusta, Maine, before joining the army medical corps. During World War I, she was stationed at Fort Riley, Kansas, developing a program to provide nutritious rations for soldiers. After her service in the army, she became a dietitian and instructor of dietetics at Massachusetts General Hospital before she was recruited by Mayo Clinic.

Initially, Mary Foley was employed by the Kahler Corporation to work in a dietary kitchen established in one of their hospitals. The lobby area was converted into a large dining room, where dietitians worked with ambulatory patients individually and in groups. Mary and a colleague projected slides with information and provided models of food and charts. They gave demonstrations on how to weigh food, cook vegetables, and wash bran to remove starch. They assisted diabetic patients as well as others who needed therapeutic diets. Dr. Will Mayo was quite impressed with the diet kitchen and asked to have the service expanded.[18]

In 1922, a colleague of Mary Foley's moved with the related physician service to Saint Marys. Mary stayed downtown and developed the Rochester Diet Kitchen in the Curie Hospital. The entire first floor was remodeled to be a restaurant with seating capacity for one hundred patients and visitors. Again, individual and group instruction was provided. By 1927, Mary had six assistants and six student interns. The Rochester Diet Kitchen was the first of its kind in the nation.[19]

Often the preliminary goal when working with patients was to dispel misinformation they had acquired about food and nutrition. One patient, for example, had been told that protein foods caused headaches and she should avoid most dairy and meats. Instead, she was told to eat one English walnut a day. Mary and her staff informed the woman that she would have to eat 109 walnuts a day to obtain enough protein.[20]

The diet kitchen staff put special foods like matzos on display so Jewish patients could see that their needs would be met. The

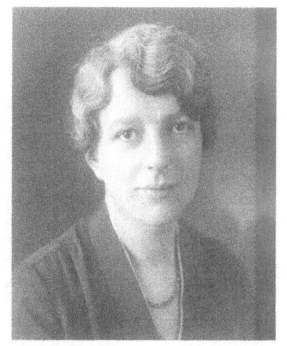

Mary Foley

dietitians also took into account the region from which the patient came so they could make recommendations of foods that would be readily available at home. Private dining rooms were provided for patients prone to seizures and those with prominent disfigurements so they could study and eat without feeling self-conscious. Diets were routinely provided for twenty to twenty-five conditions. More than five thousand patients were referred to the diet kitchen in 1930. In addition to serving patients, the kitchen provided a rich opportunity for nursing and dietary students to learn.[21]

In 1934, Mary Foley's high standard of service was recognized when she became a member of Mayo Clinic's voting staff. Created as a body when the clinic formalized its corporate structure, the voting staff consisted primarily of the permanent physicians and a few highly regarded administrators and practitioners. Mary Foley was also appointed as an assistant professor of medicine in dietetics in the Mayo Foundation Graduate School at the

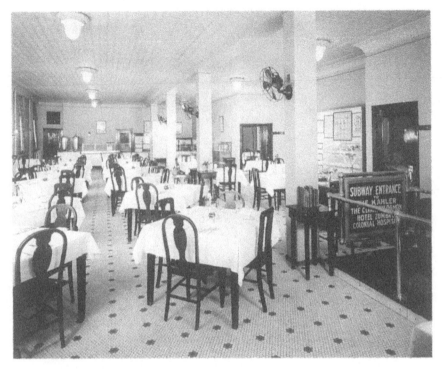

Rochester Diet Kitchen

University of Minnesota. She was active in professional organizations nationally, including serving as president of the Minnesota State Dietetics Association. Several physicians recognized her contributions by establishing the Mary Foley summer camp for diabetic children.[22]

Mary Foley's colleague Daisy Ellithorpe began work on inpatient dietetic services at Saint Marys Hospital and in 1923 was joined by Florence Hazel Smith, another nationally recognized dietitian. Soon Sister Victor Fromm assumed leadership of the dietetics department. After a decade of developing patient booklets, the dietary staff published a nationally recognized diet manual in 1932. By 1939, they were serving 65,500 special diet meals to inpatients annually. Their notoriety brought requests for internships from around the world. In 1930, they began a formal internship program, another example of Mayo's commitment to education actualized by women at the clinic.[23]

Mary Foley's career was cut short, however, when she died of metastatic cancer in 1944 at age fifty-one. Mayo Clinic issued a statement at the time of her death noting that she was a true pioneer in her field. In addition to her accomplishments in establishing the diet kitchen and related services, they noted that

> No member of our staff has earned more respect or
> more appreciation than Mary Foley. Hers was a saintly
> character, with God's loving kindness and His charity
> for all people reflected always in the beauty of her face.
> Thousands of our patients owe their health and many
> of them life itself to the ministrations, friendliness and
> devotion of this kindly, gifted teacher. Her cheerfulness
> and hopefulness also were remarkable. Stricken herself in
> the end with recurrence of malignancy, an arm painfully
> disabled, she carried on efficiently for several years with
> never a compliant. She lectured to her patients on the
> morning . . . when she left us to seek some rest with her
> family . . . her death . . . came unexpectedly to many of her
> friends. [All who knew her] will long feel deep bereave-
> ment in her loss.

Thus "closed a brilliant career in the field of dietetics."[24]

In the early 1920s, another young woman forged a unique career at Mayo Clinic. In addition to Eleanora Fry and the medical illustrators and photographers, Dr. Will Mayo sought to have a sculptor on the staff who could form three-dimensional anatomical images for presentation at meetings and exhibitions. Nellie Starkson graduated from Rochester High School in 1920 and attended Minneapolis School of Art and Design, intending to become an interior designer. Hearing about her talent, Dr. Will asked if she would be interested in becoming an anatomical sculptor if they funded her training. She agreed and soon was learning from Kenji Hayami, world famous for his wax models. In addition, she took courses in dissection and anatomy and physiology at the University of Minnesota, Johns Hopkins University, and McGill University.[25]

Nellie was very successful at her art. Her wax models were on display at the American Medical Exhibit in 1925 and in the Mayo Clinic exhibit at the Century of Progress International Exposition, a world's fair held in Chicago in 1934–35. But her work also had a lasting impact and touched patients individually. A man came to Rochester in 1968 when many of Nellie's wax models were on display in a museum in the clinic. One of the models depicted a woman with the symptoms of myxedema, also called hypothyroidism. After viewing the model and reading the associated symptoms, he immediately recognized similarities to his wife's appearance and condition. She had been suffering for some time, but no physician had been able to diagnose her problem. He immediately called his wife and insisted that she come to Rochester to be seen by a Mayo Clinic physician. She did and was diagnosed and successfully treated for myxedema. Their daughters later began showing symptoms and were similarly diagnosed and treated. The man was exuberant in his letter of gratitude, noting that the museum exhibit "changed, and perhaps saved, the life of a fine person and helped her two daughters develop normally. . . . We will forever be indebted to Mayo Clinic and the Mayo Medical Museum." Nellie, considered to be the only anatomical woman sculptor in the United States, continued in this role at Mayo Clinic until 1935, when she began working at the Chicago Field Museum. During this time, she shared an apartment with one of her sisters and enjoyed painting landscapes in her leisure. Along with many people who were called out of their careers during World War II, Nellie joined the U.S. Air Force at age forty-one and served in an aeromedical laboratory in Dayton,

Ohio. After her discharge, she moved to Florida, where she lived for many years before returning to the Rochester area to spend her retirement.[26]

Women continued to accept fellowships and join the Mayo Clinic staff in significant numbers from 1915 to the early 1930s. In addition to Dr. Stacy and Dr. Drips in gynecology, Dr. Luden was working on cancer research, Dr. Frances Ford was appointed in radiology, and several women were added in internal medicine and the department of laboratory medicine and pathology, including Dr. Winifred Ashby, whose research in blood made a major contribution.

Winifred Ashby came to Mayo Clinic in 1917 following an interesting path from London, England, her birthplace. Her family immigrated to Chicago, where she grew up and obtained a bachelor's degree from the University of Chicago in 1903. She continued her education at Washington University in St. Louis, where she earned a master's degree in biology. From 1904 to 1906, she worked on plant physiology at the University of Chicago and the U.S. Bureau of Plant Industry. She did research on infant mortality with the bureau of health in the Philippines in 1906 to 1908. In 1909 and 1910, she helped immigrants at the Northwestern University Settlement. She also taught physics and chemistry in high schools in Illinois and Missouri from 1910 to 1914. After working in laboratories at Rush Medical College and the Illinois Central Hospital in Chicago in 1916, she was accepted as a fellow at Mayo Clinic in immunology. Her mentor, renowned chemist Julius Stieglitz, wrote in support of her application for the fellowship, "Miss Ashby . . . impressed me as a woman of self-reliance, ability and good working power . . . she is bright and her painstaking persistence and steadiness in following out any line of work should head to a successful issue. That she has courage and strength is shown by the fact that she was one of the first of American women to spend a year or two in the Philippine Islands."[27]

Dr. Winifred Ashby

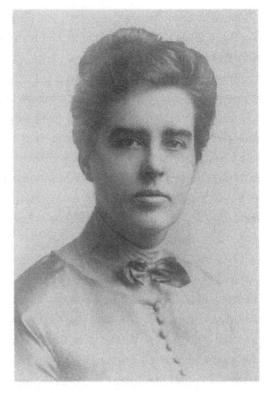

When Winifred Ashby began her work in immunology at Mayo Clinic, the blood types A, B, and O had recently been described. She developed a technique to measure the life-span of red blood cells, determining that red blood cells lasted as long as 110 days, not two to three weeks as previously speculated. This important finding provided a basis for utilizing blood transfusions to manage chronic anemia, and the technique was named "the Ashby Method," still considered one of the most important discoveries made by a Mayo Clinic researcher.

In 1921, Winifred Ashby received her PhD from the University of Minnesota; although the progressive institution had permitted women in graduate programs for some time, her diploma read "the degree of Doctor of Philosophy conferred on *him*." Dr. Ashby was appointed to the Mayo Clinic staff in the department of experimental bacteriology and experimental medicine. She continued studying anemias until she accepted a position at St. Elizabeth's Hospital in Washington, DC, in 1924. There, she managed the serology and microbiology laboratories and published the results of her studies on serologic tests for syphilis. Much of her work was done before federal funding for medical research existed, so she paid laboratory personnel out of her own salary. In the 1940s, her studies of carbonic anhydrase activity in the central nervous system were internationally recognized. Dr. Ashby lived to be ninety-two years old. Even in her last years, she remained intrigued by medical questions and was pursuing the cause of sudden infant death syndrome.[28]

After a slight dip in patient registrations after World War I, Mayo Clinic began growing again. By the mid 1920s, more than 60,000 patients registered each year and more than a third of them had surgery. Rochester had twelve hundred hospital beds and twenty-seven operating rooms solely for Mayo Clinic patients. One hundred forty rooms were dedicated to clinical laboratory procedures and research. Although hospital facilities had been expanded during this period, the clinic building, which opened in 1914, was too small. Additional space had been rented in the downtown area, but it was inefficient and insufficient. With Dr. Will Mayo's approval, Dr. Henry Plummer began planning the next Mayo Clinic building, one that would extend the capacity and ideals of group medicine.[29]

CHANGING THE GUARD

1928–1943

A new grand Mayo Clinic building opened after more than forty years of growth—but just before the inception of the Great Depression. The years that followed were challenging economically, politically, and personally. And yet, the women and men of Mayo Clinic and Saint Marys Hospital persevered even as the founders lessened their presence and eventually died, leaving a new generation to carry on, committed to the mission of alleviating human suffering.

——————

On Sunday afternoon, September 16, 1928, ten thousand people, including some from as far away as South America and Canada, gathered outside for the dedication of the new twelve-story Mayo Clinic building and carillon. The twenty-three bell, eighteen-ton carillon was specifically dedicated as a memorial to the American soldier. During the carillon performance, an airplane flew overhead, dropping five hundred red roses on the audience. The program consisted of speeches and a concert, but no tours of the new building were given. Dr. Charlie Mayo announced that due to the urgent need to begin using the facility, it would open floor by floor when ready without waiting for the entire complex to be finished.[1]

The library and reading room were moved into the twelfth floor of the new building. Maud Mellish Wilson had been designated head of the publications division, which included the library, editorial staff, and art studio. The library, which had grown substantially in

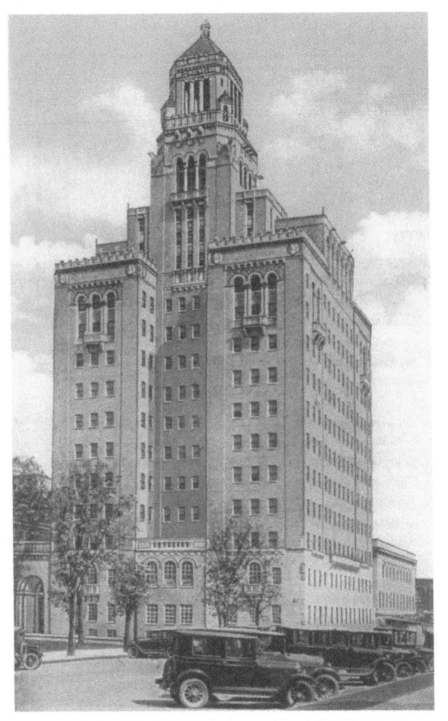

Mayo Clinic Building, 1928

the twenty years since Maud's arrival, was now staffed with full-time librarians, who provided reference services for the staff and cared for the collection of journals and 20,000 books.[2]

Maud was as busy as ever with the move into the new building and the expanding publications. In addition to reviewing nearly every paper published by Mayo Clinic staff, she initiated the publication of *The Proceedings of the Staff Meetings of the Mayo Clinic*, a summary of cases presented at the weekly staff meetings. The journal grew quickly in circulation and influence.[3]

Although Maud was admired and appreciated by many on the staff, some of her colleagues found her overbearing. She was also known to engage in heated debates with physicians over revisions to their manuscripts. The head librarian occasionally appealed to Dr. Will for additional staff and the freedom to choose her employees without interference. Dr. Will remained supportive of Maud.[4]

Maud's professional life advanced, and her personal life changed. In 1924, after seventeen years of working together, Maud and Dr. Louis B. Wilson married. Dr. Wilson had been widowed in 1920, when his wife died of arteriosclerosis, a hardening of her arteries. As head of the laboratories, Dr. Wilson was internationally recognized for many of his contributions, probably most notably for his development of the frozen section technique of slide preparation, which expedited the diagnosis of conditions during surgery, especially cancer. During his service in the armed forces during World War I, he led a successful effort to expand laboratories at military bases throughout Europe. During this time, he developed an interest in wounds caused by projectiles. He was a talented photographer and promoted the early use of photography in the Mayo practice to document operations and unusual patient conditions. He was also the first director of the graduate programs in medicine then referred to as fellowships.[5]

Maud and Louis hired Harold Crawford, who had designed Dr. Luden's carriage house and by then many other buildings in Rochester, to design their home. They built a Trenton limestone house on fifty acres of land, where they also had an apple orchard, extensive flower and vegetable gardens, and a herd of sheep to trim the grass. They preserved many of the native flowers found on the property. A darkroom was installed on the third floor for Louis's photography. A two-hundred-foot rifle range on the property allowed him to continue to study ballistics. One of the barns was used for experimental research, including the studies that Dr. Drips conducted before the clinic built facilities. They named their place Walnut Hill, and it was perhaps one of the most eclectic properties in Rochester.[6]

Drs. Will and Charlie were beginning to retire from the practice. Dr. Will, at age sixty-seven, stopped operating in the summer of 1928, several months before the new clinic building was finished. Dr. Charlie unexpectedly retired from his surgical practice a year later after suffering a retinal hemorrhage, bleeding in the vessels of one of his eyes, while he was preparing for a case. Shortly after that he experienced a mild stroke. The Mayo brothers had prepared for their retirements in the operating room and in the boardroom by hiring and mentoring extraordinary staff and by incorporating the clinic and instituting a committee consensus form of governance years earlier.[7]

Despite its success, Mayo Clinic was not immune to the Great Depression. Although a record-setting 67,800 patients were seen at the clinic the first year after the new building opened, growth was curtailed after the stock market crashed on October 24, 1929, and the impact rippled to Rochester. Patients could no longer afford to travel or pay for medical services to the same extent. The number of patients coming to the clinic the following year dropped to 42,600, two-thirds the peak of 1929. The clinic adjusted past bills and lowered their charges. Eventually, they had to cut salaries. The Saint Marys nursing program reduced enrollments to nearly half. Fewer graduates were able to find jobs; some were allowed to work at Saint Marys part-time for room and board. Some were

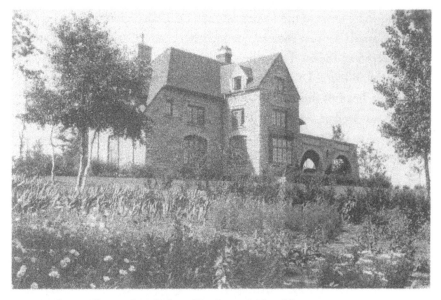

Walnut Hill, Maud Mellish and Dr. Louis Wilson's home

hired to cover the patient load previously handled by nursing students.[8]

No one was laid off in the social work department, but vacancies went unfilled and several women married and left during this period, leading to a significantly heavier workload for those who remained. Despite the 24 percent decrease in patient volumes, the staff had dropped by 50 percent, which required the director and two remaining caseworkers to exert "heroic effort" to meet patient needs.[9]

The Depression was not the only cloud in the sky. Hitler was beginning to gather influence in Germany, and possibly because of the potential for a resurgence in anti-German sentiments, or because finding space and funding for research continued to be a challenge, Dr. Georgine Luden and her companion, Betty Fitz-Gibbon, left the clinic in 1929 and moved to Victoria, British Columbia.[10]

Dr. Luden remained on very good terms with Dr. Will and Dr. Louis Wilson. They continued to correspond with her for years and share news of their work. At first, Dr. Luden did not practice in Canada because she had not taken her exams there. But in early 1942, when the head of pathology at a nearby hospital was needed in the military, Dr. Luden was awarded interim credentials and made head of the pathology laboratory. She was delighted. The lab was well organized, and the technicians' supervisor had spent a year in Rochester training, so "everything was in splendid running order." While Dr. Luden was working at the laboratory, Betty Fitz-Gibbon volunteered at the Red Cross, and together they were busy bringing their home into compliance with the blackout regulations, which was not easy because their place was "just like a big glass bird cage! Endless windows." Dr. Luden remained at the pathology laboratory until illness prevented her from continuing. She died on November 20, 1943.[11]

If circumstances in Rochester were not grim enough because of the impact of the Depression, in October 1932, Maud Mellish Wilson had exploratory surgery which revealed extensive abdominal carcinomatosis, stomach cancer. She began radiation treatments and continued to work until five weeks before her death, on November 6, 1933. Her death was described as an "irreparable loss" to the clinic.[12]

Dr. Will Mayo considered the primary founders of the clinic to be him and his brother Charlie, Dr. Henry Plummer, and Maud Mellish Wilson. He wrote at the time of her death that she was "endowed with exceptional ability, untiring perseverance, sound judgment, and indomitable courage" and "she dedicated her life to the literary development of The Mayo Clinic." Dr. Will specifically noted, "When we look back on the twenty-seven years of her faithful attention to duty, her whole-hearted cooperation with the staff in the furtherance of scientific endeavor, we realize that the educational work which she fostered is the supreme monument to the life of a great lady. We hold her in honored memory."[13]

Maud's name was engraved on the memorial wall in the Mayo

Clinic building, an honor reserved for those making the most significant contributions. Her husband, Louis, was bereft. In a letter, he mused, "I can now write, though it is still almost impossible to talk about Maud to others who loved her. Just now she fills all my waking hours . . . but I am trying to carry on as we would have together."[14]

Grace McCormick was Maud's very dear friend. They had known each other since her days in Chicago. Grace was a frequent visitor to Walnut Hill while Maud was alive. She occupied a smaller home on their property when she was in town for extended periods. Louis and Grace, grieving the loss of Maud, married the following year. Grace, who had a background in child education, established a playground and preschool program on their grounds as a tribute to Maud.[15]

On August 8, 1934, President Franklin D. Roosevelt came to Rochester to honor the Mayo brothers along with the American Legion for their great humanitarian service. After arriving by train from St. Paul, the president and other dignitaries, including Minnesota governor Floyd B. Olson, secretary of war George H. Dern, and members of the American Legion, laid a wreath at Dr. William Worrall Mayo's grave in Oakwood Cemetery. They then took a tour of Mayo Clinic, stopping at Saint Marys Hospital to greet Sister Joseph. The award ceremony took place at Soldier's Field Park, and the president's speech was broadcast by radio across the nation.

During his speech, President Roosevelt commended the Mayo brothers for the "fifty years [they] have given tireless, skillful and unselfish service here in the State and city . . . [and to the] Nation." A local artist, Edith and Charlie's daughter Louise, was commissioned by the American Legion to create bronze medallions bearing the images of her father and uncle. The individual images were then embedded in a larger bronze plaque, which was given to them.[16]

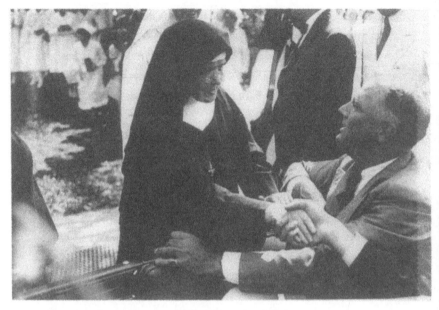

Sister Joseph Dempsey with Franklin D. Roosevelt

Afterward, the party of dignitaries was hosted by Dr. Charlie and Edith for lunch at the home they called Mayowood. Then they all drove to Wabasha, Minnesota, where they boarded Dr. Will and Hattie's yacht, the *North Star*, and cruised down the Mississippi River for the afternoon.[17]

The president's visit raised spirits and came as the impact of the Depression was beginning to lift. Edith and Hattie and their husbands were more relaxed in retirement. They owned ranch-style homes in Tucson, Arizona, where they spent portions of the winters. Although Dr. Charlie, afflicted by another stroke, was less mobile, both couples enjoyed their time in the south.[18]

In 1935, Dr. Leda Stacy, who had introduced the use of radium for treating tumors at Mayo Clinic and subsequently headed a medical section, left to join a family planning clinic at the White Plains Hospital in New York. There she was involved in giving advice about birth control to women wanting to limit the size of their families, and she helped women who wished for children but were unable to have them because of "psychological or anatomical" reasons. The family planning clinics had been well established by that time. Margaret Sanger, a nurse, opened the first family planning clinic in Brooklyn, New York, amid great resistance in 1916. After being arrested and winning challenges in court, Margaret and her associates paved the way for family planning clinics to open in increasing numbers throughout the 1920s and 1930s.[19]

Several physicians left Mayo Clinic and began practices in the East during the early thirties. Dr. Stacy had followed another Mayo physician, Dr. L. Mary Moench, who had resigned in 1932. In addition to her private practice, Dr. Moench was on the faculty of Cornell Medical College. Dr. Susan Offutt also left the clinic that year, beginning a private practice in Pittsburgh and joining the faculty of the University of Pittsburgh School of Medicine. All three of these women had been part of Dr. Stacy's section at Mayo Clinic. Dr. Della Drips, who had been in the section since 1922, declined becoming its director when Dr. Stacy left. The section was incorporated into another instead.[20]

Dr. Drips noted that Dr. Stacy's departure was a "great blow to the section." Dr. Drips had recently returned from a special course on pituitary-ovarian-uterine physiology in Berlin when Drs. Moench and Offutt left the section. After Dr. Stacy relocated, Dr. Drips and Dr. Lois Day were the only physicians remaining in the section. Dr. Stacy's patients had been seeing her for a long time, and according to Dr. Drips, "none of us could take Dr. Stacy's place.... She was greatly missed for some time." She noted that Drs. Will and Charlie were also very fond of Dr. Stacy.[21]

Dr. Drips continued to see patients and make significant contributions to research on hormones. She was frequently asked to share her "authoritative knowledge on gynecologic endocrinology" with the fellows at Mayo Clinic. After her retirement in 1949, she and Miss Jessie W. Asplin, who stepped down in 1953 after thirty-three years as a nurse anesthetist, shared a lakeside home outside of Rochester, where they enjoyed cooking and gardening.[22]

Dr. Stacy remained in close contact with her colleagues at Mayo Clinic. Shortly after her departure, Dr. Louis Wilson wrote to the authorities in New York on Dr. Stacy's behalf, recommending that she be issued a license to practice medicine in that state. In his letter he praised Dr. Stacy: "She is probably the best woman physician who has ever been on the medical staff of the Mayo Clinic. . . . During the whole time she has been with us, neither professionally or personally, has there ever been a word of criticism concerning her. She has gone to White Plains to be with friends. We would be glad to replace her in her own position at any time she would care to return."[23]

Dr. Stacy also stayed in contact with Dr. Will Mayo. She sent a letter congratulating him on his radio address in 1936, and she described the picnic she had recently held for alumni of Mayo Clinic. She noted that she had seen Daisy and Dr. Henry Plummer when they were on the Hudson River trying out a new boat. Dr. Will replied with news about staff who were ill or traveling. He closed the letter by saying, "We shall look forward to seeing you here when you make your visit in September, and we should be glad if you did not go away again. Will you please remember us kindly to Dr. Moench?"[24]

The following year, Dr. Will wrote to Dr. Stacy on behalf of Hattie, who was having trouble with psoriasis of her hands. He thanked Dr. Stacy for the hurricane lamp she sent, and he noted Hattie was having it put on the boat right away "to guide us through the first great storm that hits us. When you come out, you will see it in place. . . . Mrs. Mayo sends her love."[25]

In addition to the close personal relationships Dr. Stacy maintained in Rochester, she also retained her professional connections. Shortly after she moved to New York, she wrote to Dr. Wilson inquiring about opportunities for women to obtain internships. She reported that women graduates from Cornell Medical College were experiencing difficulty in landing positions. Dr. Stacy noted that when she graduated in 1906, only six hospitals accepted women. Subsequently, many more appointed women interns, but the recent graduates felt that the number of hospitals accepting women interns had begun to decrease.[26]

Dr. Wilson replied that according to data published in the *Journal of the American Medical Association*, all but three of the women graduates of the 1934 and 1935 classes at Cornell Medical College obtained internships. He also pointed out that internships had become increasing difficult to obtain overall, not just for women. He mentioned that sixty-eight medical colleges admitted women at the time and all were affiliated with hospitals that would typically accept their own students as interns. He observed that the subjective sentiment at Mayo Clinic about women as interns fluctuated "in correlation with the personality and attainments of the women on the fellowship staff at any given period," and he gave two specific examples. He also said that since the war, Mayo Clinic admitted the same percentage of women as were graduating from medical colleges, about four to five percent.[27]

Another woman physician also left Mayo Clinic about the same time as did Drs. Moench, Offutt, and Stacy. In 1933, Dr. Frances Ford, a radiologist, departed after twelve years at Mayo Clinic to practice in Chicago and then Oregon before settling at the Woman's Hospital in Detroit. In 1946, she went to Nanking, China, with the United Nations Relief and Rehabilitation Administration (UNRRA). Dr. Donald C. Balfour, who assumed the directorship of education after Dr. Louis B. Wilson retired from the position, wrote in support of her application to the UNRRA: "She is a fine woman, excellent radiologist, splendid character. I believe she would be well fitted for such an appointment. She is certified by the Board of Radiology and very highly regarded by specialists in that field."[28]

The result of these departures during the 1930s was dramatic. Mayo Clinic had appointed eleven women physicians to the permanent staff between 1898 and 1926. By 1935, there was only one woman, Dr. Drips, left on the permanent staff, and none would be added until 1948.[29]

Meanwhile, in life outside the clinic, Edith Mayo devoted herself to her family; she and Charlie had eight children. The next generation was leaving home. The oldest, Joseph, was lively and often needed direction. He made it through school, although he had to transfer from Princeton to finish his medical degree at the State University of Iowa in 1927. He met Ruth Rakowsky, who had come to Mayo Clinic with symptoms diagnosed as diabetes. Not long after, he wrote his parents that he wanted to marry her. Edith, concerned about her son's impulsive nature, counseled him by letter, imploring that he wait and focus on completing his medical internships before marrying, giving Ruth more time to improve her health. Edith asked Joe to "consider what is for [Ruth's] good, putting your own desires out of the question entirely, it will be the first sacrifice of your life, and will be proof to us that your love for Ruth is the enduring kind, which is the only sort that grows better with the passing years."[30]

But Joe did not follow his mother's advice and married Ruth in Joplin, Missouri, where her family lived. Edith adjusted to the situation, and she and Dr. Charlie attended the small wedding. Edith wrote to Joe's younger brother, Chuck, that Ruth was sensible and beautiful and would be a "great asset in Joe's life. Joe has something to work for that is worth while." Chuck could not attend the wedding because he was finishing his internship in Philadelphia and planning a wedding of his own.[31]

Dr. Joe and Ruth moved to Rochester after he completed his internship at Scott and White Hospital in Temple, Texas. They made their home across the lake from Mayowood in a house referred to as Bird Lodge. His older sister Edith, a graduate of Vassar College, had earned her nursing cap and pin in 1923 when she met and decided to marry Dr. Fred Rankin, a surgeon who had deployed during World War I with Unit 26 and returned to practice at Mayo Clinic. Initially they moved to Louisville, Kentucky. Later they returned to Rochester and lived in an older grand house, called White Gables, on Mayowood property until Dr. Will asked Dr. Rankin to leave the clinic due to his difficulty in getting along with other staff. It was very hard for Edith to see her daughter and grandchildren move back to Kentucky.[32]

Their artistic child, Louise, said she would never marry a doctor. Instead, she married a businessman from St. Paul, Minnesota, in 1928. When her husband became the owner of the bus company in Rochester, they moved into White Gables after Edith and her family left. The next oldest daughter, Esther, attended the Florentine School in Italy and in 1930 married a physician who decided to practice in Detroit, Michigan.

Dorothy, whose mental capacity had been affected by smallpox when she was a child, attended a boarding school owned by the Sisters of Saint Francis near Rochester into her twenties. But after watching her sisters marry, she wished to have a life of her own. Edith rented an apartment for Dorothy and hired one of her nieces, a widow with a five-year-old son, to care for her. Edith also arranged for Dorothy to have a job at Saint Marys Hospital in the pediatrics unit and provided the funds to cover her salary. After Dorothy moved, only the two youngest children remained at home.

In addition to Edith's dedication to her children, writing each of them weekly when they were in school and helping them with plans for jobs and marriage, Edith also took care of two of her sisters. In 1927, she began caring for Margaret, who came to stay at Mayowood for four months before she died of cancer. Edith's sister Dinah, who had gone to nursing school with her when they were girls, was in the next room, suffering from diabetes and pernicious anemia.

A series of tragedies would befall the Mayos and their colleagues, friends, and families during the 1930s. On December 31, 1930, Ruth and Dr. Joe adopted a baby boy they named David. During the first years of their marriage, Ruth had been pregnant three times, but the babies, all boys, were stillborn. Her difficulties were attributed to her diabetes. Dr. Charlie had been studying the challenges that diabetic women had bearing children. He encouraged them to try again. Ruth went into the hospital in her fourth month of pregnancy and remained there until August 16, 1933, when she gave birth to a baby boy delivered by cesarean section. Dr. Charlie's plan had worked and was subsequently widely replicated.

The growing family's happiness was cut short three years later on November 9, 1936, when Dr. Joe was killed in a collision with a train in Wisconsin following a duck hunting outing. After stopping for dinner and a game of poker, Dr. Joe attempted to drive home in heavy snow. He may have mistaken the train tracks for another road and inadvertently driven onto them. There was speculation that he may have been murdered because he had won a substantial amount of money at the poker table that night. As grief stricken as they were, Edith and Charlie did not push an investigation that might spur media sensationalism. The cause really did not matter—Joe was gone.

Ruth was devastated. She and Dr. Joe had lived intense lives. He was only thirty-four years old when he died; she was twenty-eight. Their sons were five and three. Edith and Louise spent time with her. Ruth and Louise both enjoyed their boats, the *Laisy Daisy* and *Blue Wren*. Ruth was a boat pilot, then an unusual skill for a woman, and she piloted the *Blue Wren* on the Mississippi as far south as New Orleans.

Many years had passed since Daisy Berkman Plummer had worked at Mayo Clinic as one of the first laboratory technicians. Daisy and Dr. Plummer had adopted a daughter and a son, who were now grown. Daisy and Henry continued to enjoy the Tudor-style home they built in 1924 and called Quarry Hill. Completion of the new Mayo Clinic building in 1928 was the culmination of

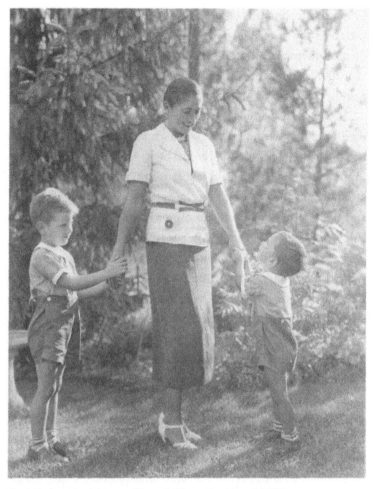

Ruth Rakowsky Mayo and her children, David and William

Henry's career in medicine and his many contributions to Mayo Clinic. After he retired from his practice and the Mayo Clinic administrative boards in 1932, they enjoyed more time on their boat. On December 31, 1936, Henry Plummer felt the symptoms of a stroke. He alerted his family and colleagues and went to bed, seeming to note the unavoidable progression of his disease with clinical interest. Daisy's husband died that night.[33]

Helen Berkman Judd, Daisy's sister and one of the other first laboratory technicians in the early days of Mayo Clinic, had been widowed the year before when her husband, Dr. E. Starr Judd, died of pneumonia on November 30, 1935, during a trip to Chicago. Dr. Judd had been the most revered surgeon at Mayo Clinic next to the Mayo brothers.[34]

In 1938, Daisy and Helen's mother, Gertrude Mayo Berkman, died. Known as Trude, she was also Dr. Will and Dr. Charlie's sister. As a young girl, she had stood by her mother's side cooking for refugees during the U.S. Dakota War in 1862. She was with the family when they came to Rochester by covered wagon. Trude was her mother's assistant for a great part of her life and then cared for her as she aged. After marrying a local veterinarian, Trude had five children, including Daisy, Helen, a daughter who married and moved to northern Minnesota, and two sons who became physicians. She had been a leader in the Magazine Club and the Rochester Civic League when it was formed.[35]

Also in 1938, Dr. Will and Hattie relinquished some of their property, including the *North Star*, their beloved "houseboat," as they called it. Others might have considered it a yacht. It was Dr. Will's favorite place to relax, and Hattie was an accomplished hostess on the water. The vessel included four staterooms for guests, two suites for the family, and an office for Dr. Will. They had owned three boats over the years, but they built the *North Star*. Hattie was said to have had a part in designing the boat, just like she had planned their home. It was 120 feet long and twenty-three feet wide. They took the *North Star* farther than their other two boats, traveling to South Carolina by way of the Gulf of Mexico, a 7,500-mile trip. They hosted dignitaries and their friends and colleagues. The Sisters of Saint Francis were frequent guests.[36]

After years of enjoying the Mississippi River by boat, Dr. Will and Hattie sold the *North Star* to the U.S. government, and it became a patrol boat off of the coast of Biloxi, Mississippi, for the duration of World War II. The proceeds went to the social services fund at the clinic to help the many patients struggling with financial burdens due to the Depression.[37]

Hattie and Dr. Will also transferred ownership of their home to the Mayo Foundation in 1938 with the intention that it be used to facilitate educational aspects of the medical practice. They moved into a smaller house constructed on their property. Dr. Louis Wilson noted that the house "has as yet unfathomed possibilities in maintaining and in further developing the goodwill and cultural and scientific ideals of all the groups who will use it." One of the Mayo surgeons paid a tribute to Hattie at the dedication, noting that she was due a "restful atmosphere" after maintaining a house that had received guests so frequently and that her dedication had allowed Dr. Will to work with "complete freedom from domestic cares and worries . . . enabling [him] to devote undivided energy and thought to his professional work."[38]

Dr. Will said, because "Mrs. Mayo and I, and our families are interested in education in the broader sense . . . we are giving our house and gardens." The house was originally planned with the intention that it be more than a place to live, but also a gathering place for clinic staff and colleagues across the country and abroad. The original plans were heavily influenced by Hattie, who demonstrated her commitment to the clinic by designing and using her home for so many functions and then ultimately giving it to the foundation.

Dr. Will noted that instruction from teachers and books are necessary to learn *what* to think, but that the great challenge is to learn *how* to think. He claimed that too much emphasis had been placed on memory tests and too little attention had been given to training that teaches applying knowledge. He and Hattie hoped their former home would be utilized to further this type of continuing education.

Tragic news reached the Mayos in Tucson during the winter of 1939. Sister Joseph had died on March 29 of an acute respiratory infection at age eighty-two. The capable Sister Domitilla had been her assistant since 1937. Sister Joseph then spent her days visiting and praying for patients, especially the poor, alcoholics, and children. She also visited many of the sisters working in the hospital who had become her good friends, including those who worked in the kitchen and bakery. She and a niece who had joined the congregation went for rides in the seven-passenger Packard that the Mayos had given them. Sister Blaise Roth had charge of the car and was a wild driver, but Sister Joseph always took the front seat so she would have a good view of the crops.[39]

An archbishop, three bishops, twenty-one priests, and as many Sisters of Saint Francis and Mayo Clinic physicians and employees as could be accommodated in the Saint Marys Hospital chapel attended the funeral mass. Surgery was suspended in the operation rooms during the service. One bishop noted Sister Joseph's courage, which endured during times of stress and uncertainty. She was remembered for her "unfailing kindness and charity, her great sympathy, fine sense of humor, sound judgment, and deep religious fervor."[40]

Dr. Will wrote, "Executives of the caliber of Sister Joseph are born, not made. Her management of the hospital has been such these many years as to give Saint Marys Hospital a unique position . . . preeminently in the regard and respect of the medical profession." He also noted that she was the best surgical assistant he ever had.[41]

Mayo Clinic physician staff revered Sister Joseph. They commissioned the creation of a bronze bust, which was dedicated in October 1939. One of the physicians said, "Sister Mary Joseph was possessed of a great love for her chosen work, a sympathetic understanding, tireless energy, indomitable courage, unusual skill as a surgical assistant and executive ability of the highest order . . . she was the guiding genius, the soul of Saint Marys Hospital."[42]

Archbishop Murray noted that the "spirit of intimacy" which existed at Saint Marys Hospital between the nursing service and medical staff contributed to the "marvelous results, which have made Rochester the medical center that it is." It would be difficult to overestimate Sister Joseph's enduring contributions.[43]

Soon after the news about Sister Joseph's death, Dr. Will decided to return to Rochester from Tucson earlier than usual because he was not feeling well. The resulting diagnosis was ominous and ironic. After a career in abdominal surgery, Dr. Will had stomach cancer. He had surgery and improved. Thinking his brother was recovering well, Dr. Charlie decided to go to Chicago for a clothes fitting. While there, he contracted pneumonia. Edith and the children gathered at his bedside, but Dr. Will was still too weak from surgery to travel. Without the benefit of antibiotics, which had not yet been developed as a medical treatment, Dr. Charlie died on May 26, 1939.[44]

The loss of Dr. Charlie was felt strongly and intimately by Edith, the family, Mayo Clinic, and the nation. But the losses were not over. Dr. Will recovered from his surgery to the point he was spending an hour or two a day in his office, but his physical health and spirits were declining. He died in his sleep the night of July 28, 1939.

Despite the losses of these pillars of Saint Marys Hospital and Mayo Clinic, the wheels were in motion to keep the institutions moving forward. Just two months later, on September 30, 1939, Sister Domitilla and the Sisters of Saint Francis broke ground for a 375-bed addition. The world-renowned medical center would persevere.[45]

Although missing their husbands immensely, Edith and Hattie continued in their roles in the community and as mothers and grandmothers. Less than a year after Dr. Charlie's death, Edith received a national honor, one that quite surprised her. She was named Mother of the Year for 1940 by the Golden Rule Foundation, a nondenominational agency dedicated to relief for needy mothers and children. Edith was selected as the mother "most representative of the best there is in womanhood." The qualities judged for the award included being a successful mother as "evidenced by the character and achievements of her children." She must also embody desirable traits: "courage, moral strength, patience, affection, kindness, understanding, home-making ability." Candidates should also have made contributions to their communities and "be equipped by nature to make friends readily."[46]

Edith received congratulations from local groups including the Mayo Clinic board of governors and the Sisters of Saint Francis, as well as from Minnesota governor Harold E. Stassen and individuals across the country. She flew to New York City with her daughter-in-law Alice and her secretary, Virginia Krause. Other family members, including her brother, Dr. Christopher "Kit" Graham, met her there. The celebration was held on Mother's Day at the Waldorf Astoria Hotel with a luncheon and radio broadcast with Sara Roosevelt, President Franklin Roosevelt's mother.[47]

In her response, Edith was modest, even suggesting that most of her success was due to her husband. She said she could think of many mothers who were more worthy than she was; she just brought up the children the best she knew. She suggested that mothers should not relegate their children's care to others and that mothers should have interests and activities outside the home, so they can bring something "fresh" to their children. Edith said that motherhood had been her whole life and she would not change anything.[48]

That same year, 1940, four years after Dr. Joe died, Ruth remarried. Her new husband was a landscape architect from California who had been a patient at the clinic. The marriage proved to be difficult, and Ruth never seemed to recover from losing Dr. Joe. On February 8, 1942, during a particularly violent argument, Ruth threw her wedding band in the fireplace and went into the

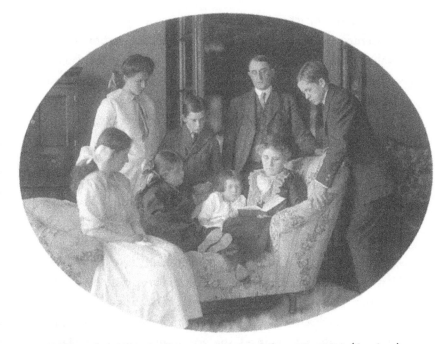

Edith reading to her family in 1912. Standing left to right: Edith (daughter),
Joe, Dr. Charlie, Chuck. Seated left to right: Dorothy, Louise, Esther.

bedroom, where she took a pistol from her bed stand and shot
herself. Joe's brother Dr. Chuck and his wife Alice rushed to help,
but Ruth died on the way to the hospital. They took Dr. Joe and
Ruth's sons, then eleven and eight years old, and raised them with
their family in the Big House at Mayowood.[49]

Ruth's death, shocking to the whole family, was especially
hard on Edith. Not long after Dr. Charlie died, since none of her
children were at home any longer, Edith had decided to move out
of the Big House and into Ivy Cottage, their first, smaller country
home at Mayowood. The Big House was more suitable for her
son Chuck and his wife Alice to raise their growing family. Edith
was without Dr. Charlie, her eldest son, and her daughter-in-law,
and another war was looming.[50]

Although the impact of the Depression was waning, World War II was gaining momentum. After the attack on Pearl Harbor on December 7, 1941, Mayo Clinic coped with the impact of the war on staff and supplies. Saint Marys Hospital nursing program reached out and accepted the transfer of Japanese nursing students who had been sent to relocation camps in the West, another example of the sisters' inclusiveness.[51]

By 1942, Edith had twenty grandchildren, seven of whom lived nearby. She enjoyed spending time with them playing cards and sharing stories. Her adopted daughter, Marilyn "Sally," joined the U.S. Women's Army Corps and was planning on getting married. Edith helped her as well as she could. By summer when her son Dr. Chuck returned from commanding military hospital units in New Guinea and the Philippines, Edith had been diagnosed with leukemia. She continued to live in Ivy Cottage and enjoyed visits from Dr. Chuck and others to hear the latest news from the clinic. As her condition progressed, she was admitted to Saint Marys Hospital, where she died on July 26, 1943. Her last days were spent being cared for in the very place she helped establish fifty-four years earlier.[52]

With Edith's death, most of the founding generation was gone. Maud's husband, Dr. Louis B. Wilson, died a few months later on October 5, 1943, of amyotrophic lateral sclerosis (ALS), two years after Lou Gehrig—also a Mayo Clinic patient—died of the disease. Hattie Damon Mayo lived until 1952, and Daisy Berkman Plummer lived to be ninety-eight years old, dying in 1976.

The new generation had taken the reins at Mayo Clinic. Edith's son, Dr. Chuck, was a successful surgeon and on the board of governors. Hattie's daughters had married Mayo Clinic surgeons and were following the example set by their mothers in supporting their families and their husband's careers.

AFTERWORD: THE LEGACY

Mayo Clinic continued to grow after Edith Graham Mayo died in 1943. The number of patients coming to Rochester increased from the temporary dip to 43,000 during the Depression to 400,000 in 2015. Since the days of the founders, Mayo Clinic has opened and affiliated with seventy-two community practices across the Midwest and opened substantial medical centers in Arizona and Florida. A total of 1.4 million patients are seen annually across all Mayo Clinic locations. They come from every state and 140 countries and from all walks of life, including U.S. presidents, the Dalai Lama, farmers, and the homeless.[1]

Each patient is given a unique registration number, continuing the system Mabel Root implemented in 1907. Today the medical record is electronic and may look quite different from the document she and Dr. Henry Plummer devised, but it still integrates all of a patient's medical history and assures the information is accessible to all members of the medical team.

The clinic building that opened in 1928 is now referred to as the Plummer Building in honor of Daisy's husband. A new clinic building, the Mayo Building, was built in 1955, and yet another new structure, the Gonda Building, opened in 2001 with a capacity of 1.6 million square feet. Many of the same design principles that Dr. Plummer incorporated in the original clinic building in 1914 and refined in the 1928 building continue to serve the purpose of supporting an efficient flow of patients through the facilities.[2]

Nursing, which began with Edith Graham Mayo as a twenty-two-year-old recent graduate, now consists of 12,000 women and men in Rochester alone who provide nationally recognized care.

The laboratory that Dr. Isabella Herb and Daisy Berkman Plummer started now employs six hundred people and performs nine million laboratory tests annually. The social work section is staffed by 149 social workers who support patients in the Rochester region, continuing the tradition started by Charlotte Bundy and her colleagues.[3]

Hattie Damon Mayo's and Maud Mellish Wilson's homes remain gathering places for Mayo staff, facilitating the exchange of ideas. Edith Graham Mayo's home, Mayowood, serves as a meeting place for Mayo personnel and is also open to the public for tours. Daisy Berkman Plummer gave her home, Quarry Hill, to the city of Rochester to become a center for the arts.

Saint Marys campus now has fifty-five state-of-the-art operating rooms and 1,350 beds, compared with the twenty-seven beds it had when Mother Alfred opened it in 1889 and twice as many as at the time of Sister Joseph's retirement. This growth in inpatient beds is remarkable given the amount of surgery that is now performed on an outpatient basis and the short length of stay needed for most hospitalizations. All of this grew out of what Mother Alfred, Sister Joseph, Sister Domitilla, and the Sisters of Saint Francis started.

The main library at Mayo Clinic is still in the same location as when Maud Mellish Wilson was there, but the collection now contains 400,000 archival volumes of books and journals and provides access to 4,300 journals electronically. In addition, librarians staff facilities at fifteen other Mayo Clinic locations. Maud started all of this from nothing. An editorial section diligently reviews papers for clarity and professionalism. The journal Maud began, now named *Mayo Clinic Proceedings*, continues to be a highly influential medical periodical throughout the world, communicating the latest clinical applications and research with a circulation of 127,000 subscribers. The medical illustrators at Mayo Clinic now work with computer-generated images but adhere to many of the same principles of illustration that Eleanora Fry utilized when she headed the art studio.[4]

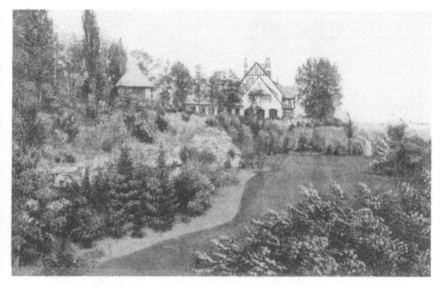

Quarry Hill, Daisy and Dr. Henry Plummer's home

The classroom portion of nursing education now occurs within colleges and universities rather than within Mayo hospitals, but Sister Joseph, Anna Jamme, and Sister Domitilla influenced many of the foundations of nursing education, and nurses continue to fulfill their clinical rotations at Mayo hospitals. The dietary and social work internships that Mary Foley and Charlotte Bundy and their colleagues started continue today.

Dr. Gertrude Booker Granger, Dr. Isabella Herb, Dr. Leda Stacy, Dr. Winifred Ashby, Dr. Georgine Luden, Dr. Della Drips, and five other women were among the first physicians at Mayo Clinic from 1898 into the 1920s. There are now 4,200 physicians and scientists at Mayo Clinic locations across the country. Those first women who practiced medicine at Mayo Clinic were true pioneers, capable and courageous.[5]

Quite simply, Mayo Clinic would not be the internationally renowned medical center it is today without the contributions made by women from the very beginning.

ACKNOWLEDGMENTS

I am indebted to a long list of family, friends, and colleagues who supported me for four years and endured listening to my stories and excitement as I uncovered these women's stories.

I am especially grateful to Sister Ingrid Peterson, who offered her expertise as a writer and historian as well as her warm friendship and persistent encouragement. Many other Sisters of Saint Francis provided guidance, including Sister Ellen Whelan, Sister Lauren Weinandt, Sister Generose Gervais, Sister Linda Wieser, Sister Kate Zimmerman, and Sister Marlys Jax. I am grateful to these sisters specifically and to the entire congregation, which consists of strong, courageous women of faith and action. Their gifts have created a legacy that will endure for many generations.

Renee E. Ziemer and the staff of the Mayo Clinic historical unit were invaluable during my research. They shared a treasure of well-organized artifacts and papers that helped me piece together these stories. They also shared their enthusiasm for Mayo Clinic's past.

The History Center of Olmsted County staff and volunteer and author Ken Allsen helped me access materials. I also made frequent trips to the Rochester Public Library, which has sparked my imagination and fed my insatiable curiosity since childhood.

Dr. Paul D. Scanlon, Johanna S. Rian, and staff of the Mayo Clinic Dolores Jean Lavins Center for Humanities in Medicine sponsored extraordinary exhibitions created by a gifted designer, Sharon L. Erdman, which brought many of these stories to life visually at Mayo Clinic.

There would be no Chapter 7 without Carole J. Stiles. While

director of social work at Mayo Clinic, she generously and enthusiastically shared tubs of materials hidden in a closet that recorded her department's history, including patient perspectives.

Many writers and teachers helped me at various points along the way on this project and others; Catherine Watson and Ashley Shelby have been especially insightful and encouraging.

Many, many friends encouraged me throughout my research and writing and listened to me talk about the book for the last four years. I especially want to thank Dr. Claire E. Bender, Dr. Gretchen A. McCoy, and M. Marsha Hall at Mayo Clinic, who were part of Mayo Clinic's history from the 1970s and with whom I had the privilege of working during my career there. Also huge thanks to my great colleagues and friends at University of Minnesota Rochester, especially Yuko Taniguchi and Bronson Lemer. Other friends who contributed along the way include Dr. Stephanie K. Carlson, Jill Caudill, Dorothea Fritz, Margaret Harwick Herrell, Bethany Krom, Dawn Littleton, and Sue Ramthun.

My siblings—Ann Garritty, Sandy Kelm, and Roger Peterson—who have tolerated my eccentricities since childhood, were also supportive, as was my favorite son-in-law, Christopher Hesby. And I would be remiss if I did not mention my faithful canine companion, Beethoven, who sat patiently next to me day after day while I read and typed.

I am also deeply grateful to editor Shannon Pennefeather and her colleagues at Minnesota Historical Society Press, who have helped these women's stories reach a broad audience. Their expertise, shared in a wonderful spirit of collaboration, made this book possible.

I was inspired by the women in my family who were also a part of Mayo Clinic's story from the early years to the present as nurses and medical secretaries: my grandmother, Pauline (Ganong) Peterson; my great-aunt, Josephine Peterson; and my mother, Marlys (Schultz) Peterson. My daughter, Kristina, continues the tradition as a nurse at Mayo Clinic today and is as innovative, courageous, and dedicated as any of the women I have written about. And thank you to my granddaughter, Harper, who as a toddler helped me rearrange the pages on multiple occasions.

Finally, thank you to my husband, Ralph, who encouraged me to write for the duration of our marriage, which ended far too soon, when leukemia took his life. His spirit, along with my father's, has been with me every step of the way.

FREQUENTLY MENTIONED WOMEN

Alfred (Moes), Mother
Founded Saint Marys Hospital

Berkman, Gertrude "Trude" Mayo
Daughter of Louise Mayo and sister to Drs. Will and Charlie

Bryant, Nell
Nurse deployed during World War I

Bullard, Florence
Nurse deployed during World War I

Bundy (Learmonth), Charlotte
Began social work

Domitilla (DuRocher), Sister
Administrator of Saint Marys Hospital 1939–49

Drips, Della
In first class of fellows; physician in women's medicine and researcher

Foley, Mary
Started dietetics for outpatients

Granger, Gertrude Booker
First woman physician to work with Mayo practice

Guthrey, Nora
Secretary deployed during World War I; Dr. Will's secretary

Joseph (Dempsey), Sister
Saint Marys Hospital Administrator 1890–1937; Dr. Will's surgical assistant

Luden, Georgine
Physician researcher in cancer

Magaw (Kessler), Alice
Nurse anesthetist known as "Mother of Anesthesia"

Mayo, Edith Graham
First formally educated nurse in Mayo practice; married to Dr. Charlie Mayo

Mayo, Hattie Damon
Married to Dr. Will Mayo

Mayo, Louise Wright
Married to Dr. William Worrall Mayo; mother of Dr. Will and Dr. Charlie Mayo

Root, Mabel
Established registration and medical records systems

Stacy, Leda
Physician head of her own section; established radium therapy

Wilson, Maud Mellish
Director of publications (library, editing, and art studio)

NOTES

NOTES TO CHAPTER 1

1. "Mayo Clinic Facts," Mayo Clinic, last modified December 2014, http://www.mayoclinic.org/about-mayo-clinic/facts-statistics.
2. Mearl W. Raygor, *The Rochester Story* (Rochester, MN: Schmidt, 1976), 1, 3, 11.
3. "Rochester's Worst Disaster, Cyclone of 1883, Swept City 50 Years Ago Today," *Rochester Post-Bulletin*, August 21, 1933, 1; "Disastrous Cyclone Struck City Sixty Years Ago Today," *Rochester Post-Bulletin*, August 21, 1943.
4. "Nun Who Came to Here in 1881 Recalls Disastrous Cyclone," *Rochester Post-Bulletin*, February 14, 1951, 8.
5. C. N. Ainslie to Burt Eaton, January 19, 1933, History Center of Olmsted County.
6. Nina C. Wagoner, personal narrative, March 13, 1944, History Center of Olmsted County.
7. Wagoner narrative.
8. "Disastrous Cyclone Struck City Sixty Years Ago Today."
9. "Mayo Boys, Hunting Sheep's Head, Caught in Cyclone 43 years ago; Horse Ran Away," *Rochester Post-Bulletin*, September 3, 1926, 3.
10. "Cyclone Hits Rochester," *Record and Union* (Rochester, MN), August 24, 1883, 3.
11. "Disastrous Cyclone Struck City Sixty Years Ago Today"; Sister Ellen Whelan, *The Sisters' Story: Saint Marys Hospital—Mayo Clinic 1889 to 1939* (Rochester, MN: Mayo Foundation for Medical Education and Research, 2002), 41–42.
12. "Cyclone Hits Rochester."
13. "Rochester's Disaster," *Rochester Post*, August 27, 1883.
14. "The Cyclone," *Record and Union* (Rochester, MN), August 31, 1883.
15. W. D. Hurlbert to John P. Finley, September 3, 1883, printed in *Rochester Record*, September 7, 1883.
16. "Once More the Cyclone Visits this County!" *Rochester Record and Union*, August 24, 1883, 1; Whelan, *The Sisters' Story*, 41–42.
17. "Rochester's Disaster."
18. W. D. Hurlbert to John P. Finley, September 3, 1883; Tom Weber, "The Tornado that Transformed Rochester," *Rochester Post-Bulletin*, August 24, 2008.

19. Helen Clapesattle, *The Doctors Mayo* (Minneapolis: University of Minnesota Press, 1941), 14–15, 126, 127.
20. Whelan, *The Sisters' Story*, 67–68.

NOTES TO CHAPTER 2

1. Mrs. William Brown Melony, "Mrs. Mayo, Wilderness Mother," *Delineator* (September 2014): 9, 46.
2. "The History of Malaria, an Ancient Disease," Center for Disease Control and Prevention (CDC), accessed December 25, 2011, http://www.cdc.gov/malaria/about/history/; Margaret Humphreys, *Malaria: Poverty, Race, and Public Health in the United States* (Baltimore, MD: Johns Hopkins University Press, 2001), 23–24.
3. Charles Dickens, *American Notes* (1842), quoted in Humphreys, *Malaria*, 31–32; Mark Twain, *Life on the Mississippi* (1883), quoted in Humphreys, *Malaria*, 33.
4. John Duffy. "The History of Asiatic Cholera in the United States," *Bulletin of New York Academy of Medicine* 47.10 (October 1971): 1152–68; John Noble Wilford. "How Epidemics Helped Shape the Modern Metropolis," *New York Times*, April 15, 2008, http://www.nytimes.com/2008/04/15/science/15chol.html.
5. Judith Hartzell, *I Started All This: The Life of Dr. William Worrall Mayo* (Greenville, SC: Arvi Books, 2004), 38.
6. Clapesattle, *The Doctors Mayo*, 18.
7. Details of the Mayos' early married life, here and in the following paragraphs, Hartzell, *I Started All This*, 18–19, 21, 31–34, 38–40.
8. Linda Peavy and Ursula Smith, *The Gold Rush Days of Little Falls* (St. Paul: Minnesota Historical Society Press, 1990), xvi.
9. Louise Mayo, "Fashionable Millinery!" *Daily Minnesotan* (St. Paul), October, 2, 1855.
10. Hartzell, *I Started All This*, 42–43.
11. Hartzell, *I Started All This*, 43, 49; Melony, "Mrs. Mayo," 9.
12. Peavy and Smith, *Gold Rush Days*, 93–102.
13. Melony, "Mrs. Mayo," 9.
14. Details on the Mayos' early years of marriage, here and below, Hartzell, *I Started All This*, 46, 48–49.
15. Details on the U.S.–Dakota War, here and below: Gary Clayton Anderson and Alan R. Woolworth, eds., *Through Dakota Eyes: Narrative Accounts of the Minnesota Indian War of 1862* (St. Paul: Minnesota Historical Society Press, 1988), 1, 8, 12–15, 19, 20; Hartzell, *I Started All This*, 43.
16. Louise Mayo's recollections of the war, here and below: Melony, "Mrs. Mayo," 46.

17. Hartzell, *I Started All This*, 64.

18. Clapesattle, *The Doctors Mayo*, 42.

19. Melony, "Mrs. Mayo," 46.

20. Clapesattle, *The Doctors Mayo*, 82.

21. Clapesattle, *The Doctors Mayo*, 173.

22. Melony, "Mrs. Mayo," 46.

23. Hartzell, *I Started All This*, 78.

24. Clapesattle, *The Doctors Mayo*, 82.

25. Hartzell, *I Started All This*, 87.

26. Homestead Church Bulletin, Rochester, MN, n.d.; Grace [last name unknown] to Isabel Farr, October 27, 1953—both Louise Wright Mayo folder, Mayo Clinical Historical Unit and Archive.

27. Melony, "Mrs. Mayo," 46; Hartzell, *I Started All This*, 96.

28. Clapesattle, *The Doctors Mayo*, 78, 81.

29. *Rochester Post*, November, 30, 1877; "Grasshopper Plagues, 1873–1877," Minnesota Encyclopedia, Minnesota Historical Society, accessed, January 5, 2012, http://www.mnopedia.org/event/grasshopper-plagues-1873-1877; Annette Atkins, *Harvest of Grief: Grasshopper Plagues and Public Assistance in Minnesota, 1873–78* (St. Paul: Minnesota Historical Society Press, 1984), 28.

30. Details about the Mayo family in Rochester, here and below: Hartzell, *I Started All This*, 97–98, 100, 101.

NOTES TO CHAPTER 3

1. Whelan, *The Sisters' Story*, 45; Sister Carlan Kraman, *Odyssey in Faith: The Story of Mother Alfred Moes* (Rochester, MN: Sisters of Saint Francis, 1990), 173–74.

2. Whelan, *The Sisters' Story*, 46; Kraman, *Odyssey in Faith*, 173–74.

3. Kraman, *Odyssey in Faith*, 175–76.

4. *Caroline and Mary Clarke* Ship Logbook, November 8, 1851, film M237, reel 107, list 1627, National Archives and Records Administration.

5. Kraman, *Odyssey in Faith*, 16, 18, 21.

6. Kraman, *Odyssey in Faith*, 16; Nicolas Gonner, *Luxembourgers in the New World*, 2nd ed., eds. Jean Ensch, Jean-Claude Muller, and Robert E. Owens, trans. Gerald L. Liebenau and Jean-Claude Muller (Esch-sur-Alzette: Editions-Reliures Shortgen, 1987), 27.

7. Gonner, *Luxembourgers in the New World*, 5, 29.

8. Whelan, *The Sisters' Story*, 19.

9. Kraman, *Odyssey in Faith*, 19, 23.

10. Kraman, *Odyssey in Faith*, 24.

11. *New York Times*, November 8, 1851.

12. Kraman, *Odyssey in Faith*, 4; Whelan, *The Sisters' Story*, 19.

13. Whelan, *The Sisters' Story*, 22.

14. Sister Ingrid Peterson, *Keeping the Memory Green: Mother Alfred and the Sisters of Saint Francis* (Rochester, MN: Sisters of Saint Francis, 2013), 4.

15. Peterson, *Keeping the Memory Green*, 4; Kraman, *Odyssey in Faith*, 35.

16. Whelan, *The Sisters' Story*, 28.

17. Father Pamfilo da Magliano quoted in Peterson, *Keeping the Memory Green*, 7.

18. Peterson, *Keeping the Memory Green*, 43.

19. *Joliet Annals* quoted in Peterson, *Keeping the Memory Green*, 8.

20. Peterson, *Keeping the Memory Green*, 9.

21. Whelan, *The Sisters' Story*, 30–31.

22. Whelan, *The Sisters' Story*, 35–36.

23. *Rochester Post*, n.d.

24. Susan B. Anthony quoted in *Rochester Post*, December 28, 1877; "Nineteenth Amendment to the U.S. Constitution: Women's Right to Vote," National Archives, accessed July 12, 2015, http://www.archives.gov/historical-docs/.

25. "Woman Suffrage," *Rochester Post*, November 2, 1877.

26. Whelan, *The Sisters' Story*, 37–38.

27. Whelan, *The Sisters' Story*, 39.

28. Details on the new hospital, here and below: "St. Mary's Hospital," *Rochester Post*, October 4, 1889.

29. Whelan, *The Sisters' Story*, 64.

30. Whelan, *The Sisters' Story*, 66.

31. Peterson, *Keeping the Memory Green*, 29.

32. Peterson, *Keeping the Memory Green*, 27.

33. "Hospital Investigation," *Rochester Post*, October 4, 1889.

34. Whelan, *The Sisters' Story*, 67.

35. Clapesattle, *The Doctors Mayo*, 253–54; Whelan, *The Sisters' Story*, 68.

36. Whelan, *The Sisters' Story*, 68–69.

37. Kraman, *Odyssey in Faith*, 177–80.

38. Judith Hartzell, *Mrs. Charlie: The Other Mayo* (Greenville, SC: Arvi Books, 2000), 15.

39. Christopher Graham quoted in Hartzell *Mrs. Charlie*, 9.

40. Neita Oviatt, "He Lived Abundantly," unpublished manuscript, box 7, Charles H. Mayo Collection, Mayo Clinic Historical Unit and Archive.

41. Harriet W. Hodgson, *Rochester: City of the Prairie* (Sun Valley, CA: American Historical Press, 1994).

42. Edith Graham Mayo quoted in Hartzell, *Mrs. Charlie*, 13.

43. Nora Guthrey, *Medicine and Its Practitioners in Olmsted County Prior to 1900* (Minneapolis: Minnesota Medicine, 1949–51), 117.

44. "Demography: Chicago as a Modern World City," Encyclopedia of Chi-

cago, Chicago Historical Society, http://www.encyclopedia.chicagohistory
.org/pages/962.html.

45. Hartzell, *Mrs. Charlie*, 17.

46. Clapesattle, *The Doctors Mayo*, 145.

47. Whelan, *The Sisters' Story*, 1–6.

48. Whelan, *The Sisters' Story*, 38–39.

49. Kraman, *Odyssey in Faith*, 198–201, 203.

50. Kraman, *Odyssey in Faith*, 213–15.

51. *Olmsted County Democrat* (Rochester, MN), December 22, 1899, quoted in
    Kraman, *Odyssey in Faith*, 215.

52. Whelan, *The Sisters' Story*, 70.

53. Whelan, *The Sisters' Story*, 71.

54. Hartzell, *Mrs. Charlie*, 23–25.

55. Hartzell, *I Started All This*, 109–11.

56. Hartzell, *I Started All This*, 110–11; Nora Guthrey, "Family Friend Tells the
    Story of Life of the Late Mrs. Mayo," *Mayovox* 3.7 (1952).

NOTES TO CHAPTER 4

1. Clapesattle, *The Doctors Mayo*, 371.

2. University of Minnesota, "Twenty-fifth Annual Commencement Program," Minneapolis, MN, June 3, 1897.

3. *Rochester City and Olmsted County Directory* (Albert Lea: Minnesota Directory Company, 1900).

4. Guthrey, *Medicine in Olmsted County*, 180–82.

5. *Northwest Journal of Medicine and Surgery* 1 (1870–81): 52–53.

6. *Northwest Journal of Medicine and Surgery* 1 (1870–81): 263.

7. *Northwest Journal of Medicine and Surgery* 1 (1870–81): 270.

8. *Northwest Journal of Medicine and Surgery* 1 (1870–81): 381–82.

9. *Northwest Journal of Medicine and Surgery* 1 (1870–81): 382–84.

10. *Northwest Journal of Medicine and Surgery* 1 (1870–81): 382–84.

11. Regina Morantz-Sanchez, *Sympathy and Science: Women Physicians in
    American Medicine*, 2nd edition (Chapel Hill: North Carolina University
    Press, 2000), 51–53, 58, 137.

12. William Worrall Mayo quoted in Clapesattle, *The Doctors Mayo*, 131.

13. Clapesattle, *The Doctors Mayo*, 132.

14. Guthrey, *Medicine in Olmsted County*, 181.

15. Guthrey, *Medicine in Olmsted County*, 183.

16. Leonard G. Wilson, *Medical Revolution in Minnesota: A History of the Uni-
    versity of Minnesota* (St. Paul, MN: Midewiwin Press, 1989), 565.

17. Morantz-Sanchez, *Sympathy and Science*, 51–53, 58, 137.

18. Morantz-Sanchez, *Sympathy and Science*, 51–53, 58, 137.

19. Morantz-Sanchez, *Sympathy and Science*, 249; Thomas Neville Bonner, *To The Ends of the Earth: Women's Search for Education in Medicine* (Cambridge, MA: Harvard University Press, 1992), 156, 169.

20. Morantz-Sanchez, *Sympathy and Science*, 262.

21. "Married at Noon," *Olmsted County Democrat* (Rochester, MN), February 16, 1900, 1.

22. Gertrude Booker Granger, "Analysis of 13,000 Cases for Errors of Refraction," *Lancet*, May 15, 1913.

23. "Moved Yesterday: The Drs. Mayo, Stinchfield and Graham Now in their New Quarters—Weber & Heintz, Ditto," *Olmsted County Democrat* (Rochester, MN), December 7, 1900.

24. Jeffery E. Nelson and Steve F. Wilstead, "Alice Magaw (Kessel): Her Life In and Out of the Operating Room," *Journal of American Association of Nurse Anesthesia* 77.1 (2009): 12–13; Hartzell, *Mrs. Charlie*, 15.

25. Jeanne Pougiales, "The First Anesthetizers at the Mayo Clinic," *Journal of American Association of Nurse Anesthetists* 38.3 (1970): 237.

26. Pougiales, "The First Anesthetizers," 235.

27. Evan Koch, "Alice Magaw and the Great Secret of Open Drop Anesthesia," *Journal of American Association of Nurse Anesthesia* 67.1 (1999): 33–34.

28. Nelson and Wilstead, "Alice Magaw (Kessel)," 1, 14; Clapesattle, *The Doctors Mayo*, 431.

29. Robert A. Strickland, "Isabella Coler Herb: An Early Leader in Anesthesiology," *Anesthesiology Analgesia* 80: 600–604.

30. Strickland, "Isabella Coler Herb," 600–604.

31. Daisy Berkman Plummer, "Reminiscences of Dr. Henry Plummer," interview by Clark W. Nelson; Daisy Berkman Plummer, "Mrs. Henry S. Plummer, Miss Mabel Root, and Dr. F. A. Willius," interview by William Holmes, 1960—both Daisy Plummer Collection, Mayo Clinic Historical Unit and Archive.

32. Plummer interview, "Mrs. Henry S. Plummer, Miss Mabel Root, and Dr. F. A. Willius."

33. Strickland, "Isabella Coler Herb," 600–604.

34. Charles M. Guthrie, "91-Year-Old Pioneer Looks Back—and Ahead," *Rochester Post-Bulletin*, 1969, History Center of Olmsted County; Henry S. Plummer letters to Daisy Berkman Plummer, Daisy Plummer Collection, Mayo Clinic Historical Unit and Archive.

35. "Pretty Home Wedding: Miss Daisy Berkman and Dr. Henry D. Plummer Take Marriage Vows," undated newspaper article, Daisy Plummer Collection, Mayo Clinic Historical Unit and Archive.

NOTES TO CHAPTER 5

1. Dr. William J. Mayo to Maud Mellish, January 1, 1907, Mellish-Wilson Collection, Mayo Clinic Historical Unit and Archive.

2. Dr. William J. Mayo to Maud Mellish, February 12, 1907, Mellish-Wilson Collection, Mayo Clinic Historical Unit and Archive.

3. "Demographics," "Art," and "Music," Encyclopedia of Chicago, Chicago Historical Society, http://www.encyclopedia.chicagohistory.org.

4. Clapesattle, *The Doctors Mayo*, 518–20.

5. Wilson, "In Memoriam, Maud Mellish Wilson," *Supplement to Proceedings of the Staff Meetings of the Mayo Clinic* 8.51 (1933).

6. Mrs. D. J. Rogers to Louis B. Wilson, November 18, 1933, box 2, Mellish-Wilson Collection, Mayo Clinic Historical Unit and Archive.

7. Wilson, "In Memoriam, Maud Mellish Wilson."

8. Ernest J. Mellish quoted in Wilson, "In Memoriam, Maud Mellish Wilson."

9. Maud Mellish, *The Writing of Medical Papers* (Philadelphia: Saunders, 1922).

10. Wilson, "In Memoriam, Maud Mellish Wilson."

11. Mabel Root, interview, Henry Plummer Collection, Mayo Clinic Historical Unit and Archive.

12. Root interview.

13. Root interview.

14. Leda Stacy, "Twenty-eight Years at the Mayo Clinic," unpublished manuscript, 1957, Leda Stacy Collection, Mayo Clinic Historical Unit and Archive.

15. Stacy, "Twenty-eight Years at the Mayo Clinic."

16. "Wedded at Mayo Home," *Olmsted County Democrat* (Rochester, MN), May 29, 1908.

17. "Wedded at Mayo Home."

18. "Mid Ferns and Roses," *Post and Record* (Rochester, MN), May 29, 1908.

19. Nelson and Wilstead, "Alice Magaw (Kessel)," 15.

20. Nelson and Wilstead, "Alice Magaw (Kessel)," 15; V. Thatcher, *History of Anesthesia with Emphasis on the Nurse Specialist* (Philadelphia: J. B. Lippincott Co., 1953), 57.

21. Alice Ellis to author, February 20, 2014; "Invalid Woman, 73 Years Old, Dies of Burns," *Rochester Post-Bulletin*, May 23, 1932.

22. Magazine Club Collection, Mayo Clinic Historical Unit and Archive.

23. Clapesattle, *The Doctors Mayo*, 471–73; Hartzell, *I Started All This*, 149–51.

24. Hartzell, *Mrs. Charlie*, 34.

25. Mayo Clinic Division of Publications, *A Sketch of the History of the Mayo Clinic and the Mayo Foundation* (Philadelphia: Saunders, 1926), 19.

26. "On the Auction Block: Highest Bidder for Former Mayo Home Will Get Lots of History," *Rochester Post-Bulletin*, November 11, 1986, 5C; Hartzell, *Mrs. Charlie*, 25–27.

27. Hartzell, *Mrs. Charlie*, 26.

28. "Historic Mayowood Mansion: A Pictorial Guide," Olmsted County History Center, 2000.

29. Undated newspaper article, Administrative Scrapbook, Mayo Clinic Historic Unit and Archive; Flo Becker, "The Women's League of Rochester, Minnesota: History and Development," unpublished manuscript, Olmsted County History Center.

30. "Resignation as Tendered," *Rochester Post and Record*, December 4, 1918.

31. Undated newspaper article, Administrative Scrapbook, Mayo Clinic Historic Unit and Archive; Mary Dillion Foster, "Rochester Women's Civic League" and "Emma Potter Allen," *Who's Who Among Minnesota Women* (St. Paul: M. D. Foster, 1924).

32. *Sketch of the History of the Mayo Clinic*, 31.

33. *Sketch of the History of the Mayo Clinic*, 22, 24–25.

34. "The Mayo Clinic Building Is Formally Opened," *Rochester Daily Bulletin*, October 11, 1912, 1.

NOTES TO CHAPTER 6

1. "Mayo Clinic Building Formally Opened," 1.

2. "Formal Opening of Clinic Building Attracts Hundreds of People Friday," *Rochester Post and Record*, March 7, 1914.

3. "Formal Opening of Clinic Building"; Richard Olding Beard, "The Mayo Clinic Building at Rochester," *Journal-Lancet* reprint, August 15, 1914.

4. Clapesattle, *The Doctors Mayo*, 531.

5. Thomas B. Magath, presentation, July 7, 1971, Thomas Magath Collection, Mayo Clinic Historical Unit and Archive.

6. *Sketch of the History of the Mayo Clinic*, 84.

7. Rebekah A. Dodson, "Eleanor Fry: Illustrator to the Mayo Brothers," unpublished manuscript, June 1989, Eleanora Fry Collection, Mayo Clinic Historical Unit and Archive, 6; book review, *Practical Cystoscopy and the Diagnosis of Surgical Diseases of the Kidneys and Urinary Bladder* by Paul M. Pilcher, *American Journal of Surgery* 25.12 (1911): 407–8.

8. Information in this and the following paragraphs from Dodson, "Eleanor Fry: Illustrator to the Mayo Brothers," 8, 9, 14, 15.

9. "Olmsted County Public Health History," unpublished document, Olmsted County Public Health Department; "Achievements in Public Health 1900–1999: Control of Infectious Diseases," United States Center for Disease Control and Prevention (CDC), last modified July 30, 1999, http://www.cdc.gov/mmwr/preview/mmwrhtml/mm4829a1.htm.

10. Stacy, "Twenty-eight Years at the Mayo Clinic."

11. Christopher Graham to Robert D. Mussey, January 23, 1918, Christopher

Graham Collection, Mayo Clinic Historical Unit; Stacy, "Twenty-eight Years at the Mayo Clinic."

12. James E. Thompson to William J. Mayo, January 9, 1913, box 64, W. J. Mayo Collection, Mayo Clinic Historical Unit and Archive.

13. "Doctor Luden, Former Researcher Here, Dies in Canada," *Rochester Post-Bulletin*, November 22, 1943.

14. Harold H. Crawford, "Peace and War," unpublished manuscript, Harold Crawford Collection, History Center of Olmsted County.

15. Hartzell, *I Started All This*, 158; Clapesattle, *The Doctors Mayo*, 473; "Statue Ceremony," *Olmsted County Democrat* (Rochester, MN), June 4, 1915, 2–3.

16. "Mrs. Louise Mayo Passes Away at Age of Ninety Years After Life of Real Service," *Rochester Bulletin*, July 15, 1915.

17. "Mrs. W. W. Mayo Passes Away," *Rochester Post and Record*, July 16, 1915, 5.

18. Crawford, "Peace and War."

19. Ken Allsen, *Master Architect: The Life and Works of Harold Crawford* (Rochester, MN: History Center of Olmsted County, 2014).

20. Allsen, *Master Architect*.

21. Georgine Luden to Harold H. Crawford, December 31, 1918, Harold Crawford Collection, History Center of Olmsted County.

22. Thomas Farr Ellerbe, *The Ellerbe Tradition: Seventy Years of Architecture & Engineering* (Minneapolis, MN: Ellerbe, Inc., 1989), 16; Clapesattle, *The Doctors Mayo*, 476–77.

23. *Sketch of the History of the Mayo Clinic*, 146–52.

24. Helen Baldwin to Louis B. Wilson, March 9, 1921, Wilson Collection, Mayo Clinic Historical Unit and Archive; Della G. Drips, "Memoirs," unpublished manuscript, April 21, 1958, Drips Collection, Mayo Clinic Historical Unit and Archive.

25. Arlene Keeling, *The Nurses of Mayo Clinic* (Rochester, MN: Mayo Foundation for Medical Education and Research, 2014), 34.

26. Clapesattle, *The Doctors Mayo*, 565–66.

27. "Pioneer Descendent Dies at 89," *Rochester Post-Bulletin*, December 1977.

28. Harry Harwick, letter of recommendation for Nora Guthrey, Nora Guthrey Collection, Mayo Clinic Historical Unit and Archive; *Rochester Post-Bulletin*, March 1918, Nora Guthrey file, History Center of Olmsted County.

29. Wilson, *Medical Revolution in Minnesota*, 217–18.

30. D. D. Getchell, *History of Base Hospital 26* (Minneapolis: Getchell, 1920); unidentified newspaper article, Unit 26 Collection, Mayo Clinic Historical Unit and Archive.

31. Getchell, *History of Base Hospital 26*, 14–15, 34; Susan Sheehy, "U.S. Military Nurses in Wartime: Reluctant Heroes, Always There," *Journal of Emergency Nursing* 33.6 (2007): 557.

32. Nell Bryant Crenshaw, interview by Meg Diessner, 1973, John Crenshaw Collection, Mayo Clinic Historical Unit and Archive.

33. Nell Bryant to Mrs. Charles Durham, August 14, 1918, Nell Bryant Collection, Mayo Clinic Historical Unit and Archive.

34. Nell Bryant to Mrs. Charles Durham, February 23, 1919, Nell Bryant Collection, Mayo Clinic Historical Unit and Archive.

35. Nell Bryant Crenshaw interview.

36. Virginia Simons Wentzel, *Sinere et Constanter 1906–1970: The Story of Saint Marys School of Nursing* (Rochester, MN: Mayo Foundation for Medical Education and Research, 2006), 166; New York City newspaper clipping, September 9, 1918; Hardwicke Nevin, "Soissons," with handwritten dedication—both Saint Marys Hospital Historical Archive.

37. Florence Church Bullard to Sister M. Julie, August 1, 1961, Saint Marys Hospital Historical Archive.

38. Mary T. Sarnecky, *A History of the U.S. Army Nurse Corps* (Philadelphia: University of Pennsylvania Press, 1999), in Keeling, *Nurses of Mayo Clinic.*

39. "Welcome our Boys," Nora Guthrey file, History Center of Olmsted County.

40. "The Deadly Virus: The Influenza Epidemic of 1918," National Archive and Records Administration, accessed March 24, 2015, http://www.archives. gov/exhibits/influenza-epidemic/; Clapesattle, *The Doctors Mayo,* 569; Philip K. Strand, *A Century of Caring, 1889–1989: Saint Marys Hospital of Rochester, Minnesota* (Rochester, MN: Saint Marys Hospital, 1989), 38.

41. *Sketch of the History of the Mayo Clinic,* 31.

NOTES TO CHAPTER 7

1. Charlotte Bundy Learmonth, "Early Day Memories: Department of Medical Social Work Service, Mayo Clinic, May 1921–July 1925," unpublished memoir, Social Work Collection, Mayo Clinic Historical Unit and Archive.

2. Learmonth, "Early Day Memories."

3. "Ida Maude Cannon," *The Social Welfare History Project,* 2014, accessed August 23, 2015, http://www.socialwelfarehistory.com/people/cannon-ida-maude/.

4. *Sketch of the History of the Mayo Clinic,* 94.

5. Charlotte Learmonth's documentation, here and below: Learmonth, "Early Day Memories"; George M. Higgins, "Methodist Hospital History," unpublished manuscript, Social Work Collection, Mayo Clinic Historical Unit and Archive, 2.

6. Charlotte Bundy Learmonth, speech given to Magazine Club at Kahler Hotel in Rochester, MN, March 12, 1923, Social Work Collection, Mayo Clinic Historical Unit and Archive.

7. "Here Is Your Chance to Help a Worthy Cause, So Get Busy," *Rochester Post and Record,* May 29, 1921; "Hospital Social Service is Planning Extensive Library," *Rochester Post and Record,* May 22, 1921.

8. Higgins, "Methodist Hospital History," 10–12.

9. Learmonth, "Early Day Memories, 5; "Annual Report of Section of Medical Social Service: February 1, 1923 to February 1, 1924," Social Work Collection, Mayo Clinic Historical Unit and Archive.

10. Margaret Rogers to George M. Higgins, n.d., Social Work Collection, Mayo Clinic Historical Unit and Archive.

11. Blanche Peterson, "Medical Social Work with Tuberculous Patients at the Mayo Clinic," *Hospital Social Service* 17 (1928): 29–35; notes on treatment cases, here and below: Charlotte Bundy (Learmonth), "Medical Social Work," unpublished manuscript, January 9, 1924, Social Work Collection, Mayo Clinic Historical Unit and Archive.

12. Bundy (Learmonth), "Hospital Social Services Bulletin No. 9," March 1, 1923, Social Work Collection, Mayo Clinic Historical Unit and Archive.

13. "Social Significance of Gonorreha and Syphilis," Minnesota State Conference of Social Work, presentation by unnamed Mayo Clinic social worker, May 24, 1928, Social Work Collection, Mayo Clinic Historical Unit and Archive.

14. "Medical Social Service Annual Report: February 1, 1923 to February 1, 1924," 17–18.

15. Juliet Eisendrath, untitled manuscript, n.d., Social Work Collection, Mayo Clinic Historical Unit and Archive; "Our History," B'nai Israel Synagogue, last modified July 6, 2007, www.bnaiisrealmn.org/aboutus/history.

16. Details about the occupational therapy program, here and below: "The Rochester Methodist Hospital Associated Professional Services: B- Occupational Therapy," unpublished manuscript, Social Work Collection, Mayo Clinic Historical Unit and Archive.

17. "Hospital Social Service Bulletin," January 20, 1923, Social Work Collection, Mayo Clinic Historical Unit and Archive.

18. "The Rochester Methodist Hospital Associated Professional Services," 6 (Miss Gladys Pattee), 7.

19. "Hospital Social Services Bulletin No. 13," January 8, 1923, Social Work Collection, Mayo Clinic Historical Unit and Archive.

20. F. Stuart Chapin to Louis B. Wilson, January 14, 1926, Social Work Collection, Mayo Clinic Historical Unit and Archive.

21. Charlotte Bundy (Learmonth) to Harry J. Harwick, May 20, 1922, Social Work Collection, Mayo Clinic Historical Unit and Archive; "Social Services History: 75 Years," brochure, 2011, Social Work Collection, Mayo Clinic Historical Unit and Archive.

22. "Medical Social Service at the Mayo Clinic Scrapbook," Social Work

Collection, Mayo Clinic Historical Unit and Archive; Learmonth, "Early Day Memories," 11–12.

23. "Priscilla Keely to be Senior Staff Member of Social Service," *Mayovox*, June 20, 1953, Social Work Collection, Mayo Clinic Historical Unit and Archive; "Medical Social Service at the Mayo Clinic Scrapbook."

24. Higgins, "Methodist Hospital History."

25. Clapesattle, *The Doctors Mayo*, 586–89.

26. "Mishap During Blackout Fatal to Interpreter," *Rochester Post-Bulletin*, December 10, 1951, 10; photo, Mayo Clinic Historical Unit and Archive.

NOTES TO CHAPTER 8

1. Strand, *A Century of Caring*.

2. Gunther W. Nagel, quoted in Whelan, *The Sisters' Story*, 85; I. H. Dar, et al., "Sister Mary Joseph Nodule: A Case Report with Review of Literature," *Journal of Research Medicine Science* 14.6 (2009): 385–87.

3. *Sketch of the History of the Mayo Clinic*, 25–29.

4. Strand, *A Century of Caring*, 43.

5. Description of opening celebration, including quoted remarks, here and below: "Opening of the New Surgical Pavilion of St. Mary's Hospital," *Rochester Post-Bulletin*, May 12, 1922.

6. Dr. Louis Wilson and Reverend W. W. Bunge remarks, brochure, Saint Marys Hospital Archive.

7. Sister Joseph Dempsey, "Hospital Economy," Saint Marys Hospital Archive.

8. Strand, *A Century of Caring*, 75; "A Souvenir of Saint Mary's Hospital," brochure, 1922, Saint Marys Archive, 29.

9. Strand, *A Century of Caring*, 76.

10. Wentzel, *Sinere et Constanter*, 83.

11. William J. Mayo, address to the Alumni of Saint Marys Hospital, May 27, 1919, Sister Joseph Collection, Mayo Clinic Historical Unit and Archive.

12. Helen Clapesattle, interview with Sister Domitilla DuRocher, March 20, 1934; Helen Clapesattle, "Data Pertaining to Saint Mary's School of Nursing April 1934," unpublished manuscript, box 1, Clapesattle Collection, Mayo Clinic Historical Unit and Archive.

13. Wentzel, *Sinere et Constanter*, 82–83, 94, 95–97; "New Auditorium is Opened with Organ, Orchestra Recital," *Rochester Post-Bulletin*, n.d., Sister Joseph Dempsey Collection, Mayo Clinic Historical Unit and Archive.

14. Wentzel, *Sinere et Constanter*, 87–88.

15. Wentzel, *Sinere et Constanter*, 88; Sister Domitilla DuRocher interview; Whelan, *The Sisters' Story*.

16. Keeling, *Nurses of Mayo Clinic*, 49.

17. "Rochester State Hospital Graduate Nurses Reunion 1892–1943," brochure, History Center of Olmsted County; Wentzel, *Sinere et Constanter*, 47.

18. Russell M. Wilder, "Recollections and Reflections," *Perspectives in Biology and Medicine* (1958): 244.

19. Wilder, "Recollections and Reflections," 244.

20. *Staff Meetings of the Mayo Clinic* (Rochester, MN: Mayo Clinic, 1931), 459.

21. *Staff Meetings of the Mayo Clinic*, 460–61.

22. "Mary Foley 51 Years Old, Dies in East," *Rochester Post-Bulletin*, April 8, 1944.

23. Whelan, *The Sisters' Story*, 130–31.

24. "Minutes of Council," Mayo Clinic, Mary A. Foley Collection, Mayo Clinic Historical Unit and Archive; "Mary Foley Dies in East."

25. "Rochester Native Is Only Woman Anatomical Sculptor in America," *Rochester Post-Bulletin*, January 9, 1943.

26. Carl B. Philips to Robert C. Roesler, March 23, 1977, Mayo Clinic Historical Unit and Archive; "Nellie Starkson, 78, Ex-Illustrator, Dies," *Rochester Post-Bulletin*, October 16, 1981, 22.

27. "Winifred Ashby," *Physicians of the Mayo Clinic and Mayo Foundation with Portraits* (Philadelphia: W. B. Saunders, 1927); on Dr. Ashby's biography, here and below: Virgil F. Fairbanks, "Doctor Ashby of Virginia: An Admiring Profile," *The Mayo Alumnus* (1975), Ashby Collection, Mayo Clinic Historical Unit and Archive.

28. "Dr. Winifred M. Ashby, Bacteriologist, Dies," *Washington Post*, July 26, 1975, B3.

29. *Sketch of the History of the Mayo Clinic*, 30–31, 90.

NOTES TO CHAPTER 9

1. "Guest Carillonneur Lauds Quality of Bells in Clinic," *Rochester Post-Bulletin*, September 17, 1928, 3; "Flower Shower," *Rochester Post-Bulletin*, September 17, 1928, 1; Clapesattle, *The Doctors Mayo*, 797.

2. *Sketch of the History of the Mayo Clinic*, 107.

3. Louis B. Wilson, "A Woman Pioneer in a New Profession, Medical Editing," *Supplement to Proceedings of the Staff Meetings of the Mayo Clinic* 8.51 (1933).

4. Megan Cole, "Maud the Mayo Years," unpublished manuscript, Mellish-Wilson Collection, Mayo Clinic Historical Unit and Archive; F. S. C. James to William J. Mayo, October 17 and November 11, 1916, box 8, William J. Mayo Collection, Mayo Clinic Historical Unit and Archive.

5. Wilson, "A Woman Pioneer"; Mrs. L. B. Wilson Dies Suddenly at Home Here," *Rochester Post-Bulletin*, July 6, 1920; Clark W. Nelson, "Louis B. Wilson: Historical Profile," *Mayo Proceedings* 69.4 (1994).

6. Matthew D. Dacy, "The Wilson House on Walnut Hill," pamphlet, Walnut Hill Collection, Mayo Clinic Historical Unit and Archive.

7. Charles W. Mayo, *Mayo: The Story of My Family and Career* (New York: Double Day, 1968), 80–81.

8. "Patient Registrations and Counts 1921–1943," Registration Collection, Mayo Clinic Historical Unit and Archive; William J. Mayo, address to Mayo Clinic staff, Rochester, MN, August 11, 1930, box 8, William J. Mayo Collection, Mayo Clinic Historical Unit and Archive; Wentzel, *Sinere et Constanter*, 38–39.

9. Higgins, "Methodist Hospital History," 14.

10. Georgine Luden to Louis B. Wilson, August 10, 1924, and January 25, 1925, box 14, Wilson Collection, Mayo Clinic Historical Unit and Archive.

11. Georgine Luden to Louis B. and to Grace Wilson, January 31, 1942, box 14, Wilson Collection, Mayo Clinic Historical Unit and Archive; "Dr. Luden, Former Researcher Here, Dies in Canada," *Rochester Post-Bulletin*, November 22, 1943.

12. Wilson, "A Woman Pioneer."

13. R. Beard interview with William J. Mayo, boxes 5, 6, Clapesattle Collection, Mayo Clinic Historical Unit and Archive; Wilson, "A Woman Pioneer."

14. Louis B. Wilson to Miss Pitman, box 2, Mellish-Wilson Collection, Mayo Clinic Historical Unit and Archive.

15. "Grace McCormick," unpublished manuscript, Wilson Collection, Mayo Clinic Historical Unit and Archive.

16. Franklin D. Roosevelt, "Address Delivered at Rochester, Minnesota," August 8, 1934, *The American Presidency Project*, accessed June 15, 2015, http://www.presidency.ucsb.edu/ws/?pid=14737; Hartzell, *Mrs. Charlie*, 92.

17. "August 8, 1934," *Franklin D. Roosevelt Day by Day*, Franklin D. Roosevelt Library, accessed June 15, 2015, http://www.fdrlibrary.marist.edu/daybyday/daylog/august-8th-1934/.

18. Hartzell, *Mrs. Charlie*, 108.

19. "Dr. Stacy, Retiring, Is Honored at Tea," unnamed newspaper, Stacy Collection, Mayo Clinic Historical Unit and Archive; "Achievements in Public Health 1900–1999."

20. *Physicians of the Mayo Clinic*, 99, 1061; Stacy, "Twenty-Eight Years at the Mayo Clinic."

21. Drips, "Memoirs."

22. Katharine Smith, "Della G. Drips, M.D.," Album of Women in Medicine, *Journal of the American Medical Women's Association* 10 (1955): 29; "Jessie Asplin, Anesthetist for Thirty-Three Years, Has Brief Comment on Career, Six Months Retirement," *Mayovox*, June 20, 1953, 2.

23. Louis B. Wilson to Harold L. Rypis, October 4, 1935, Stacy Collection, Mayo Clinic Historical Unit and Archive.

24. Leda J. Stacy to William J. Mayo, June 11, 1936; William J. Mayo to Leda J. Stacy, June 20, 1936—both box 67, William J. Mayo Collection, Mayo Clinic Historical Unit and Archive.

25. William J. Mayo to Leda J. Stacy, October 1, 1937, box 67, William J. Mayo Collection, Mayo Clinic Historical Unit and Archive.

26. Leda J. Stacy to Louis B. Wilson, March 29, 1936, box 15, Wilson Collection, Mayo Clinic Historical Unit and Archive.

27. Louis B. Wilson to Leda J. Stacy, April 4, 1936, box 15, Wilson Collection, Mayo Clinic Historical Unit and Archive.

28. Donald. C. Balfour, telegram to E. P. Morh, Ford Collection, Mayo Clinic Historical Unit and Archive.

29. Mayo Clinic, "Rochester Women Appointed to Staff 1898 through 1980."

30. Edith Mayo quoted in Hartzell, *Mrs. Charlie*, 78.

31. Details on Edith Mayo's life and family, here and below: Hartzell, *Mrs. Charlie*, 78, 80–81, 82, 89, 90–91, 95, 100–101.

32. Mayo, *The Story of My Family and My Career*, 83.

33. Clapesattle, *The Doctors Mayo*, 709.

34. Clark W. Nelson, *Mayo Roots: Profiling the Origins of Mayo Clinic* (Rochester, MN: Mayo Foundation for Education and Research, 1990), 132.

35. "Sister of Mayo Brothers, Here 75 Years, Dies," *Rochester Post-Bulletin*, July 22, 1938.

36. Matthew D. Dacy, *A Passion for the River: Mayo and the Mississippi* (Rochester, MN: Mayo Foundation for Medical Education and Research, 2004).

37. Dacy, *A Passion for the River*.

38. Comments at dedication, here and below, "Mayo Foundation House, Once Home of Dr. William J. Mayo, Dedicated to Good of Mankind," *Rochester Post-Bulletin*, September 24, 1938.

39. Whelan, *The Sisters' Story*, 154–55, 156.

40. *Saint Marys Alumnae Quarterly*, May 1939, 8, Saint Marys Hospital Archive.

41. William J. Mayo quoted in *Saint Marys Alumnae Quarterly*, May 1939, 8.

42. Julius H. P. Gauss quoted in "Honor Memory of Sister, Hospital Head Many Years," *Rochester Post-Bulletin*, October 26, 1939.

43. Archbishop Murray quoted in "Honor Memory of Sister."

44. Clapesattle, *The Doctors Mayo*, 711.

45. Sister Mary Brigh, "Medical History in Minnesota; A Symposium: Saint Marys Hospital," lecture given at the 57th Annual Meeting of the Medical Library Association, June 2–6, 1958, Rochester, MN.

46. "Mrs. Charlie H. Mayo Named 'American Mother for 1940,'" *Rochester Post-Bulletin*, April 17, 1940.

47. "American Mother Flies East to Receive Title," *Rochester Post-Bulletin*, May 9, 1940.

48. "Motherhood Has Been Whole Life, American Mother for 1940 Says," *Rochester Post-Bulletin*, April 29, 1940.
49. Mayo, *The Story of My Family and My Career*, 188–89.
50. Hartzell, *Mrs. Charlie*, 111.
51. Wentzel, *Sinere et Constanter*, 56.
52. Hartzell, *Mrs. Charlie*, 119–20.

NOTES TO AFTERWORD

1. "Patient Registrations and Counts 1921–1943"; "Mayo Clinic Facts," Mayo Clinic, accessed July 9, 2015, http://www.mayoclinic.org/about-mayo-clinic/facts-statistics.
2. "Leslie and Susan Gonda Building, Mayo Clinic, Rochester, Minnesota," Healthcare Design, last modified August 31, 2003, http://www.healthcare designmagazine.com/article/leslie-susan-gonda-building-mayo-clinic-rochester-mn.
3. "Laboratory Medicine and Pathology in Minnesota," Mayo Clinic, accessed July 9, 2015, http://www.mayoclinic.org/departments-centers/laboratory-medicine-pathology/minnesota/overview/specialty-groups/clinical-core-laboratory-services; Carole Stiles, Director of Mayo Clinic Social Work, email to author, July 8, 2015.
4. "About Mayo Clinic Libraries," Mayo Clinic, accessed July 9, 2015, http://www.mayo.edu/library/about; "Mayo Clinic Proceedings 2014 Impact Factor," Mayo Clinic, accessed July 9, 2015, http://www.mayoclinic proceedings.org/pb/assets/raw/Health%20Advance/journals/jmcp/IF.pdf.
5. "Mayo Clinic Facts."

INDEX

Page numbers in *italics* indicate illustrations.

PICTURE CREDITS

Unless otherwise noted, all photographs are used by permission of the W. Bruce Fye Center for the History of Medicine, Mayo Clinic, Rochester, Minnesota, including photographs provided by the Saint Marys Hospital Archives.

Images pages 87, 113, 145, and 164, from author's collection.

Image page 106, used with permission of Mayo Foundation for Medical Education and Research, all rights reserved.

Image page 183, used by permission of the History Center of Olmsted County.

The text of *Women of Mayo Clinic* has been set in Arno Pro, a typeface designed by Robert Slimbach. Arno is a meticulously crafted face in the tradition of early Venetian and Aldine book typefaces, and is named after the Florentine river which runs through the heart of the Italian Renaissance.

Book design by Wendy Holdman